Mental Health Services Today and Tomorrow

PART 2

Perspectives on policy and practice

Edited by

CHARLES KAYE
Mental Health Services Consultant

and

MICHAEL HOWLETT
Director, The Zito Trust

Radcliffe Publishing
Oxford • New York

Radcliffe Publishing Ltd
18 Marcham Road
Abingdon
Oxon OX14 1AA
United Kingdom

www.radcliffe-oxford.com
Electronic catalogue and worldwide online ordering facility.

British Library Cataloguing in Publication Data

A catalogue record for this book is available from the British Library.

ISBN-13: 978 184619 262 3

Typeset by Pindar New Zealand (Egan Reid), Auckland, New Zealand
Printed and bound by TJI Digital, Padstow, Cornwall, United Kingdom

Mental Health Services
Today and Tomorrow

PART 2

Perspectives on policy and practice

**Books are to be returned on or before
the last date below.**

Contents

Preface

The progenitor of this book was a survey we carried out into the status, including successes and failures, of England's Mental Health Trusts. We describe the origins and outcomes of that survey in our Introduction. The questions posed by the survey – and the absence or incompleteness of answers on key topics – convinced us that a more extensive treatment was appropriate. But how should we go about that?

We wanted to look forward to trace and anticipate change in mental health services and to try to assess the impact both of developments in the field of care and treatment and of the implications of new organisational change. But we sought to achieve this not principally by our own knowledge and analysis, but by turning to those involved in services at all levels – to draw upon their experience to give a fuller picture of today and to help sketch in tomorrow. It was important to us to balance academic scrutiny with personal involvement, to reflect national trends and local endeavours.

Thus, for example, we deliberately juxtaposed a personal account of one man's journey through mental illness against the emergence of a new national initiative which will affect the whole country involving the treatment of hundreds of thousands of individuals at a cost of millions of pounds. It is our own view that to fail to value the reality and validity of personal experience when reviewing the pattern of care is the equivalent of building without foundations. The essential touchstone of successful care and treatment is the effect on individuals; too often, in our experience, the management of mental health services focuses on targets and totals and loses sight of its responsibility to users, carers and staff. A welter of slogans, strategies, brands and initiatives can fail to describe what happens to patients in the sub-standard psychiatric intensive care unit, to the individuals who fall between the compartmentalised services, and to the ill and inarticulate who can be shoehorned into predetermined patterns of services for the convenience of the system or the neatness of the organisation.

Consequently we have looked for detailed scrutiny – and one which reflected what users, practitioners and academics observed and experienced. Using the themes and topics identified by our survey, we commissioned chapters from a wide range of contributors asking them to describe the present and to anticipate and predict future changes, opportunities and threats. We chose contributors on the basis of their expertise and directed them towards key topics that we considered central to the future provision of care. We took pains to achieve the balance we have described. We also wanted to reach out beyond the island to take some soundings from mainland Europe. What is happening elsewhere? How might that affect our future here? Just as some contributors describe very personal experiences, so others explore a quite uncertain future, speculating and extrapolating.

From all our contributors we looked for a reasoned balance between success and problems, between observation and prophecy. We have avoided both the fatuously optimistic and the doomsayers. Above all, we invited them to 'write it as they see it'. We feel that the resulting collection of accounts gives a wide-ranging and valuable assessment of mental health services in England today.

We did, however, make a conscious editorial decision not to explore forensic mental health services in any depth (although we refer in 'Harnessing the flow' to the funding of this part of the service). One of the seminal works in the field (*Forensic Psychiatry*, edited by Gunn and Taylor, first published in 1993) is being extensively revised and will be published in 2009.

Our goal in assembling and editing these contributions has been to depict realistically the current service, to outline sympathetically its features and flaws and to suggest where future emphasis needs to be placed, both locally and nationally, to make significant improvements and, above all, to make it more responsive to the needs of users and carers.

We've arranged the material in two parts. Part 1 focuses on experiences of receiving and offering care and on the realities of providing services at a practical and local level. It is an account of frontline life in today's mental health services. In Part 2, we take much more of a helicopter view, reviewing policy and practice from national and European perspectives. The two approaches are, of course, interdependent and interlinked and both should be explored.

Our own chapter, 'Harnessing the flow', concentrates on what seem to us the most important messages that our survey highlights. Our contributors have identified a number of specific proposals that we consider would significantly improve the current service. One curious phenomenon that struck us in the task was that for all the national target-setting, organisational reshaping and the deluge of guidance, mental health services seem to lack personality; it is, in some contexts, closely defined but as a national player, curiously amorphous and passive. It would be encouraging to think that as Foundation Trust status becomes the norm, attention could be paid to the goal of creating an effective lobby representing all those personally involved in the service, a lobby that could help bring about change based on the evidence and experience of those directly involved.

Perhaps these books and their contributors might represent a significant step towards that destination.

Charles Kaye
Michael Howlett
April 2008

List of contributors

Jonathan I Bisson is a Clinical Senior Lecturer in Psychiatry at Cardiff University. He developed his interest in traumatic stress as a psychiatrist in the British Army. His research interests are in the effectiveness of early interventions following trauma and interventions to treat early symptoms and psychological predictors of the development of post-traumatic stress disorder (PTSD). He has published over 50 papers and book chapters on PTSD and related subjects. He is the President-Elect of the European Society for Traumatic Stress Studies, and chairs the Liaison Psychiatry Faculty for the Welsh Division of the Royal College of Psychiatrists. He recently co-chaired the development committee for the National Institute for Health and Clinical Excellence guidelines for PTSD.

John Bowis is Conservative Member of the European Parliament for London. He is the Spokesman for the EPP-ED Group on the Environment, Public Health and Food Safety Committee and serves on the Foreign Affairs Committee, Palestine Delegation and ACP EU Assembly. He has been the Parliament's Rapporteur on a range of policy areas, including Health and Poverty Reduction in Developing Countries, the European Centre for Disease Control and Mental Health. Between 1997 and 1999 John was International Policy Adviser to the World Health Organization's Collaborating Centre at the Institute of Psychiatry in London. From 1983 to 1997 he was the Member of Parliament for Battersea, serving as Minister for Health and Minister for Transport.

Tom Burns is Professor of Social Psychiatry at the University of Oxford. He was Professor of Community Psychiatry at St George's Hospital in London. He qualified from Cambridge University and Guy's Hospital, London, and trained in Psychiatry in Scotland and London. His research interests are predominantly health services research in community psychiatry, particularly trying to understand the components of complex interventions and the nature of the therapeutic relationship. He has written three books: *Assertive Outreach: a manual for practitioners* (2002), *Community Mental Health Teams: a guide to current practices* (2004) and *A Very Short Introduction to Psychiatry* (2006), all published by Oxford University Press. He was awarded the CBE in 2006 for services to mental healthcare.

Sarah Ellix works for Leicester City Council and has a keen interest in equality, diversity and human rights. Within the Adults and Housing Department at Leicester her role assists development of equality research and initiatives to benefit service users, providers and employees. Sarah's work cuts across the equality/human-rights spectrum, including specific work around race. Recent research has developed particular interests in dual inequalities faced by people accessing mental health services, compounded by lived experience of racism/discrimination. Her research priorities are to drive forward change and to help meet the current and future needs of Leicester's diverse population.

Simon Francis was until recently a policy adviser on disability employment strategy in the Department for Work and Pensions. He is currently seconded to the National Social Inclusion Programme working on benefit and employment policy for people with mental health needs. His research has included exploring the dynamics of economic activity in deprived areas, and he has recently completed some ethnographic research in the north-east, looking at how policy impacts on various stakeholders. He has also studied the psychosocial influences on worklessness, and has published research for the Health Development Agency on the relationship between health and work.

Jonathan Hill was educated at Leighton Park School, Reading, and then at the Royal Free Hospital School of Medicine, training in General Medicine, Homoeopathy and General Practice before commencing Psychiatry at the Mid-Wales Hospital in Talgarth. In 1995, after further training in Psychiatry at Cardiff and St George's Hospital, London, he was appointed Consultant in Adult and Old Age Psychiatry in Brecknockshire. Since 2000, with the closure of the Mid-Wales Hospital, he has been working as an Old Age Psychiatrist in Brecknockshire and Radnorshire. He has an interest in liaison Psychiatry and Dynamic Psychotherapy. He lives near Brecon with his wife and family.

Sarah Hill is the Head of Arts Therapies and Vocational Services Manager at North London Forensic Service where her role focuses on education and work experience projects as well as the arts therapies. She co-ordinates the implementation of a social inclusion model. For the last three years she has been seconded part-time to the National Social Inclusion Programme as the Business and Communications Manager. Sarah is a trustee of The Zito Trust.

Michael Howlett graduated in Law from Cambridge University and, after a period of teaching, joined the therapeutic staff at Peper Harow in Surrey, working with emotionally damaged adolescents and young offenders. He worked for the national High Security Psychiatric Service with Charles Kaye before becoming Director of The Zito Trust in 1994 which is now based in Hay-on-Wye. He has contributed a number of articles and book chapters on mental health and community care policy.

Charles Kaye graduated from Manchester University and trained in hospital management with the King's Fund in London. He held a variety of management posts in the National Health Service before being appointed in 1989 Chief Executive of the national High Security Psychiatric Service. Currently he is involved in social housing and in the provision of homes and employment for young people. He was awarded an OBE in 1996. He has edited and written books on the arts in healthcare, the management of high-security services, and on race and culture in secure psychiatric settings.

Michael Maher was Deputy Director at Peper Harow, a residential therapeutic community for adolescents. He has been Chair of the Trustees of The Zito Trust since its inception in 1994. Until recently he worked in a developmental and consultative role in providing residential and multi-agency resources in a local authority children's department. He trained at the Institute of Group Analysis in London, and is currently pursuing further training in systems-centred therapy. He now works freelance as an organisational consultant and psychotherapist with particular interests in staff groups, conflict resolution, building teams that work, and mentoring managers in high-risk positions.

Wendy Maycraft Kall studied Political Science and Public Administration at Hull University and Uppsala University in Sweden, and is a qualified accountant and a member of the Chartered Institute of Public Finance and Accountancy. She has previously been employed by the National Audit Office, carrying out financial evaluations of central government programmes and by the Chartered Institute of Public Finance and Accountancy, training public-sector managers. She is currently employed by the Department of Government at Uppsala University where she lectures in comparative public administration and social policy. Her current research interests are public-sector professions and comparative welfare policy reforms.

Alan Maynard is Professor of Health Economics at the University of York. He was Founding Director of the Centre for Health Economics at York and has been involved in National Health Service management since 1983, and Chair of York Foundation Trust Hospitals since 1997. He has Honorary Doctorates from the Universities of Aberdeen and Northumbria, and is Adjunct Professor at the Centre for Health Economics Research and Evaluation of the University of Technology, Sydney, Australia. He has worked as a consultant for a variety of national and international agencies, including the World Bank and the World Health Organization. He has written and edited a dozen books and published extensively in management and professional journals.

David McDaid is Research Fellow in Health Policy and Health Economics at LSE Health and Social Care and the European Observatory on Health Systems and Policies, both at the London School of Economics and Political Science. Currently he is co-ordinator of the EU-supported Mental Health Economics European Network and he has also acted as a consultant on mental health policy to a variety of governmental, public and voluntary agencies, including the World Health Organization and the European Commission.

Gerald O'Mahony graduated from University College Cork and trained in Psychiatry in Cardiff and London. He works as an Old Age Psychiatrist in East London and has been a Consultant at St Bartholomew's and Homerton hospitals since 1994. Gerald is the Clinical Lead for Old Age Psychiatry Services in the City and Hackney locality of East London and the City Mental Health Trust and has worked with colleagues to establish a fully integrated Community Mental Health Team with local authority partners.

Zoë Robinson worked in forensic services in west London before going on to manage community supported housing (mental health and ex-offender projects) provided by Stonham Housing Association in south London. The Social Exclusion Unit (SEU) seconded Zoë onto their mental health project to provide advice to the policy team on frontline issues and to develop policy. Zoë stayed on with the SEU to develop the factsheet, *Action on Mental Health*, on behalf on the National Institute for Mental Health in England/Care Services Improvement Partnership where she works as Delivery Manager leading on Housing and Criminal Justice.

Swaran P Singh is Professor of Social and Community Psychiatry at the University of Warwick and Honorary Consultant Psychiatrist for the East Birmingham Early Intervention Service. He trained as a psychiatrist at PGI Chandigarh, India, and was a lecturer and consultant in Nottingham before moving to St George's University of London where he developed the ETHOS early intervention service. His research interests include early psychosis, cultural and ethnic influences in mental health and health services evaluation.

Cathy Street is a freelance health researcher and consultant. She has published widely in a number of areas, including Tier 4 inpatient services, mental health services for young people with learning disabilities, gender-based differences in mental health, play as a means of promoting mental health, supporting young people excluded from school and developing user involvement. From 2000 to 2006, Cathy was the Research Lead for Young Minds, the children's mental health charity, managing the charity's national research projects *Where Next?* (new ways of delivering inpatient services) and *Minority Voices* (the acceptability and accessibility of mental health services for young people from black and minority ethnic groups).

Kala Subbuswamy is currently working as a Planning and Service Development Officer for Adult Mental Health at Leicester City Council. She has a background in psychology and has been active on a range of issues, including anti-racism, the environment and human rights. She has worked within the mental health field in Leicester for the last 10 years, and has a particular interest in the issues of recovery, empowerment and equality. She is a mental health survivor, and is part of a community time bank run by and for survivors in Leicestershire.

Christine Vize has been a consultant in general adult psychiatry for 12 years. She also works as Director for New Ways of Working (NWW) with the Avon and Wiltshire Mental Health Partnership Trust, and as Associate Director for New Ways of Working with the Care Services Improvement Partnership (CSIP). She led one of the first national pilots for NWW in mental health in her Trust, and her CSIP role involves working with many different stakeholders to implement NWW in Mental Health Trusts. She is a member of the National Steering Group on NWW and chairs one of its sub-groups and a working party.

Acknowledgements

The editors would like to thank the following for their invaluable support at various stages in the preparation of the book: Hilary Burch, Ella Chidgey, Mary Crawford, Margaret Cudmore, Alan Franey, Brenda Goddard, Deborah Hart, Vivien Norris, Malcolm Rae, John Wilderspin and Deborah Williams. They would also like to thank Radcliffe Publishing for commissioning the book and Gillian Nineham and her colleagues for their editorial guidance and advice throughout.

We are also grateful to the various individuals and organisations who gave their permission to reproduce materials, including photographs, artwork, extracts and poems.

The Heritage Model in Chapter 5 is reproduced with permission from the copyright holder Hilal Barwany on behalf of Leicester City Council.

Chapter 6, 'Race and mental health: there is more to race than racism' was originally published as an article in the *British Medical Journal* (*BMJ* 2006; **333**: 648–51) and is reprinted in its entirety under licence granted by the BMJ Publishing Group Ltd.

to Vivien, Oscar, Oliver and Martha

I'm nobody! Who are you?
Are you nobody, too?
Then there's a pair of us – don't tell!
They'd banish us, you know.

EMILY DICKINSON 1830–86

Introduction

CHARLES KAYE and MICHAEL HOWLETT

In 2005, under the aegis of The Zito Trust, we carried out a survey across all the English mental health trusts. We wanted to establish a record of how the country's mental health service had developed since its reconfiguration into largely stand-alone organisations which the *National Health Service Plan* of 2000 had initiated.

We considered that the major change presaged by that plan needed a scrutiny and consideration that had up to now been absent. We published the results of the survey, and our analysis of the significant findings, in our report, *Today and Tomorrow: better services for mental health?*[1] Of course, it was a mixed picture. In some areas, both in service and geographical terms, there was much to be lauded; in other respects, however, there were real concerns expressed by Trusts about the effectivenesss, range and financing of their services.

It was clear to us that what the Trusts' responses depicted needed exploration in more depth. Our survey, and their response, produced a useful snapshot describing and suggesting major contours – but the picture was necessarily a very broad one. We wanted to take the findings of the survey and to use them as the basis for a deeper consideration of issues identified as being central to future patterns of the provision of care and support. To do this we approached a deliberately wide range of contributors, asking them – on specifically selected topics which arose from the survey material – to outline present practice and experience, and to look forward.

This produced a rich harvest which could usefully be divided under two broad headings: the experience of the individual in receiving and participating in care and treatment; and the evaluation of policy and strategy related to national and European mental health services. *Mental Health Services Today and Tomorrow Part 2: perspectives on policy and practice* comprises these wider reviews, while our companion volume, *Mental Health Services Today and Tomorrow Part 1: experiences of providing and receiving care*, concentrates on personal experiences within mental health services as user, carer, provider and professional.

Each book stands in its own right as a lively and thought-provoking examination of mental healthcare today in England (with some important additional material in this volume describing the development of services in Europe). Each volume looks at difficulties, quandaries and problems – and suggests solutions and ways forward. In their overall scope the books are complementary and interlinked; together they offer a wide-ranging analysis of treatment and care. The experiences thus shared and the future outlined go to the very heart of current provision. Important questions are asked which need answers if the service as a whole is to match aspirations and expectations which have emerged from the major changes that have taken place over the past forty years. The gradual disappearance of the water towers marks the past ebbing away. Whether the future will redeem the ambitions and well-intentioned pledges of a new world focused on equality, respect, tolerance and the individual very much depends on our willingness to face the realities and make the choices outlined by our contributors.

Yet another review of the National Health Service (NHS) has been announced by yet another Secretary of State for Health. This review is to deliver a report before the 60th anniversary of the NHS in 2008. A major test of its value, and of the commitment to user-centred care, will be whether, amid the hurly-burly of acute care, it takes on board the real needs in mental health service provision which our two volumes so cogently describe.

REFERENCE

1 Kaye C, Howlett M. *Today and Tomorrow: better services for mental health?* Hay-on-Wye: The Zito Trust; 2005.

CHAPTER 1

Harnessing the flow

CHARLES KAYE and MICHAEL HOWLETT

THE CURRENT

Across the landscape of English public services flows the Amazon that is the National Health Service (NHS): its tributaries reach into every area and influence domestic and political life on a daily basis. It stretches from fertility to finality, sweeping along colds and cancer, phobias and psychopathy: its availability dominates local debates and its organisation, and reorganisation, is the enduring preoccupation of politicians of all hues. Despite 60 years of turbulence about funding, about clashes between politicians and the medical establishment and about central diktat versus local clamour, it remains in full spate, nationally accepted as an essential feature of today's, and tomorrow's, society.

Clearly it has changed continuously since 1948 and that change, as elsewhere in society, has accelerated in pace. While the carapace and the supportive rhetoric surrounding it has a gnarled and almost totemic presence, new forms are emerging which presage change on a scale not previously imagined. Curiously this public process of change has been visible and widely advertised but hardly recognised. Generations of politicians have struggled with the need to control and direct a service that swells by social osmosis, sucking in the needs of a population that increasingly looks for medical solutions to relieve difficulties – with doctors and a pharmaceutical industry that are just as eager and dedicated to providing those solutions. The resulting monolith – 8.2% of gross domestic product,[1] 1.3 million employees (in 2004)[2] – seems nationally unmanageable, spilling over in a thousand places, uneven and erratic.

Over the last 20 years a new national philosophy has developed – in an

unspoken and, of course, unacknowledged alliance between different governments during that time.

This could be said to have started with Roy Griffiths[3] and his recommendation
of general management, to have moved through the purchaser/provider split,
and to have come to full fruition in the current description[4] of public service
reforms which seek to:

➤ 'combine top-down approaches of inspection, regulation and targets
➤ with horizontal pressure from competition and contestability
➤ and bottom-up incentives of choice and voice
➤ supported by improvements in capability and capacity
➤ ... to create a "self improving system"'.

In practical terms for the NHS, this means the overt separation of all those
elements that provide healthcare (progressively to become Foundation
Trusts), the heavily fertilised introduction of competition from independent
healthcare providers and the creation of a national network of commissioners
who will buy the best value healthcare according to nationally set standards.
Or as the same document[5] describes it (in *hospital* terms):

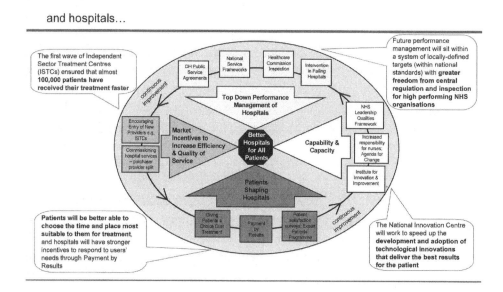

FIGURE 1.1 *Policy review: public services,* January 2007. © Crown copyright.
Reproduced with permission from Cabinet Office, Prime Minister's Strategy Unit.

So the monolith is deconstructed by separating the planning, buying and monitoring powers from the responsibility for providing. The former remains the task of government (representing the taxpayers) while the latter becomes a devolved plurality where market forces will come into play sorting out the weak and the inefficient. (Interestingly the Scottish model cleaves to 14 Health Boards responsible for planning *and* delivery of all healthcare.)

> '. . . we are likely to see the NHS evolving into a network rather than an institution: more "ecosystem" than "army".'
>
> **Stevens S. *Crosscurrents*. 50th Anniversary Edition. London: NHS Institute for Innovation and Improvement; 2006.**

This is the clear and unambiguous goal of the political leaders supported by their praetorian guard, the managers who obediently lead their cohorts onto the next target. However, all the indications suggest that the vision (rapidly becoming a reality as the first group of Foundation Trusts – including several mental healthcare providers – rather carefully flex their competitive muscles) has yet to be recognised or accepted by the NHS staff groups – who will have to make it work – or by the general public whose focus remains not the national philosophy but the local provision. Further it needs to be appreciated that this new model is essentially geared to the provision of acute healthcare and acute illness: note that the diagram above refers explicitly to 'hospitals', the behemoths of the NHS. The questions we want to ask are simple. Firstly, in practical terms how does this new analysis apply to mental healthcare? And secondly, what evidence is there that it will improve the nation's mental health?

TURBULENCE

Before we can respond to these questions, we need to describe key elements of change and conflict in the world of mental healthcare which have a major influence on that service and national opinion.

In one area, mental health has been a pioneer, setting a trend which politicians hope that acute care will follow (even if with a great deal of kicking and screaming). The exodus from the Victorian institutional model of mental healthcare has been dramatic (not just in England but throughout western Europe): the number of inpatient psychiatric beds in England has reduced from 131 825 in 1978, to 77 628 in 1988–89, to 33 000 in 2001–02.[6] In 2005–06, the figure was 29 802.[7] The new Care in the Community approach quickly ran into considerable problems and has been extensively revamped.

But the institutions themselves are now literally being built over, becoming in many places the location for new housing estates.

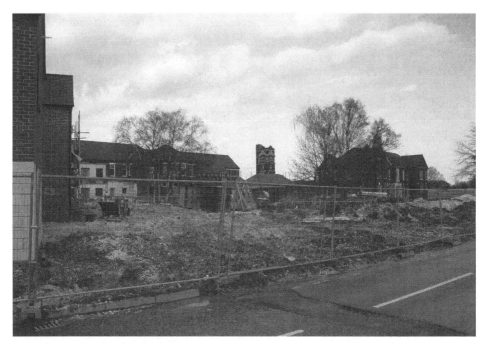

FIGURE 1.2 Park Prewett Hospital, Hampshire. Constructed between 1913 and 1916 to accommodate 1300 patients. The water tower is between the ward block and main entrance and new housing is being constructed on the left of the picture.

This de-institutionalisation, however, has exceptions: significantly the provision of secure psychiatry beds has nearly doubled in a decade, from 1557 in 1996 to 2807 in 2006.[8] Over that period secure psychiatric beds have risen from 4% of the total available to 9.4%. In the same period the prison population has risen from 45 000 (1993) to 80 000 (2006)[9] and is still rising. And while transcarceration may not be explicitly established, the dramatically high incidence of mental illness and mental disorder in the prison population has been.[10] Similar trends have been noted in several other European countries – particularly The Netherlands, Germany, Sweden and Spain.[11]

   Running alongside this massive reorientation of mental health services – and literally of many of its recipients – has been an awkward, conflicting and contentious public debate. The stigma attached to any form of mental illness has long been evident and is well illustrated elsewhere in our companion volume, *Mental Health Services Today and Tomorrow Part 1: experiences of providing and receiving care* (cf. chapters by Hegarty and O'Brien, Campbell, and Pelendrides). Much laudable effort has been invested nationally and locally to inform and educate and to counter this prejudice. Some ground has been gained by hard work and persistence, although almost daily the negative is expressed.

'Microchips for mentally ill planned in crime shake-up'

Daily Telegraph, **17 January 2007**

A survey by the Scottish Executive, however, in 2005,[12] showed an encouraging trend of better understanding and greater tolerance. This ambivalence is repeated in the 2007 survey on *Attitudes to Mental Illness* where positive responses on questions of mental illness declined compared to earlier surveys.

Nevertheless, the painstaking work of sharing and explaining is often eclipsed by the surge of fear that the reporting of a violent incident involving mental illness can release. A random stabbing on the underground or in Richmond Park speaks with greater volume and more authority than an appeal to understanding and humanity. And the Government's determined fierceness in confronting and punishing crime in many respects amplifies the volume and confirms the authority. Thus, not unusually, government's public pronouncements and attitudes – in all sincerity – broadcast different messages which compete and conflict. It may be understandable for Walt Whitman to say:

> 'Do I contradict myself?
> Very well then I contradict myself.
> (I am large, I contain multitudes.)'

From: 'Song of Myself'

But governments work on a national canvas with greater impact – and contradictions at the centre breed greater confusion!

Essentially we still live in a society which is antipathetic, frightened, suspicious and even contemptuous of mental illness, and ever ready to condemn, anathematise and even criminalise it. The experience of mental illness does not in the wider context carry with it the sympathy (or the funding) accorded to cancer sufferers or sick children and recovery does not generate the feel-good factor that, say, a successful transplant offers.

So, as we survey the turbid stream, these are our key observations:
➤ carried along with the rest of the NHS, mental healthcare is being reshaped – providers segregated and competition anticipated

➤ a highly regulated, centrally driven pattern of service has established uniform and multifarious targets with a new standard service provision to achieve them

➤ in the public arena, stigma and fear still dominate the spectators' view of mental illness; despite – or perhaps because of – its high incidence, mental illness remains ostracised

➤ mental health services have not yet fully internalised/digested the move from institution to community.

SHOOTING THE RAPIDS

The NHS has rarely enjoyed tranquillity; controversy has been both midwife and godfather. But the present time seems particularly tumultuous and as always in the public health debate when the going gets tough, it gets even tougher for mental health services. Our survey in 2005[13] revealed real concerns about finance and the availability of funds to further improvements. This note is becoming more dominant: as has always historically been the case, when the acute services go into deficit, one pocket to raid is the mental health budget. Mental Health Trusts as far apart as Nottinghamshire and Hampshire recorded in 2005–06 substantial levies they had to return to Primary Care Trusts (PCTs) to meet acute sector deficits. Public service finances are amazingly complicated, as Michael Maher describes them elsewhere in this book:

> Financial and managerial processes in the NHS are famously Byzantine in their obscurity and cumbersomeness; those of local authorities aspire to match them in these qualities.

A recent monthly financial report to a Mental Health Partnership Trust ran to 30 pages of text and charts! In addition current discussions about 'disinvestment' between newly aggregated PCTs and Mental Health Trusts anticipate cuts, however they are presented. Surveys[14,15] by Rethink in 2006 suggested that £30 million had been cut from Trusts' mental health budgets in 2005–06 with the prospect of a further £37 million to follow. The Sainsbury Centre Review[16] painted a similar picture. However, targets and expectations remain unchanged, thus generating additional pressures.

The new patterns for delivering mental healthcare have been carefully and extensively documented (e.g. *Community Mental Health Teams: implementation guide*[17]). Advice/instruction may be given on teams, caseloads and working practices but the issuing of such material – itself a destabilising cascade – does not transform one clinic, let alone a national service. Elsewhere in this book Dr Christine Vize describes the redefinition of the role of the consultant psychiatrist, but the establishment of teams as a new basis and the relinquishing of familiar territory is far from complete – and probably not understood by clinical colleagues in other settings. The hierarchy of professions in mental healthcare, dating back to the all-powerful medical superintendent, may be in the process of change but the flux – inevitable as it may be – creates further complications. The rearrangement of working practices may seem common sense but the undercurrents it conceals represent some of the most difficult and delicate areas in the service where professional standing and interdisciplinary rivalry are not management theory but everyday reality.

One feature of mental health services has been the emergence of the voice of the public – whether that is the service user, the carer or, in some cases, the victim. In different contexts these all articulate their needs, aspirations and dissatisfactions. Officially these are welcomed – ours is a consumer, customer-oriented culture; better informed, we seek better service and real responses to our complaints and needs. The mental health world pullulates with pressure groups and one consistent feature of government review of public service provision has been to establish the 'users' as an integral part of each service, citing such devices as:

➤ giving users a choice/personalisation
➤ funding following users' choices (individual budgets)
➤ engaging users through voice and co-production (representation in decision-making).

Such approaches are welcomed by users, nationally and locally, and our survey found considerable enthusiasm in Trusts for pursuing these ideas. And, of course, a stake for the public is built into the constitution of Foundation Trusts with an open membership and a council of governors. The deeper involvement of users in aspects of managing and delivering the service has had successes. But expectations, once aroused, characteristically expand and demand more. Today's first steps with users on committees or appointment boards, or being 'consulted', are unlikely to be satisfying for long. Deeper involvement – as opposed to well-meaning 'tokenism' – will be far more demanding for both users and service providers.

When the issue of 'choice' in mental health provision is properly addressed, there will be considerable readjustment called for. In many parts of the country Trusts are monopoly suppliers and have very limited awareness of, or enthusiasm for, what choice for consumers entails. Major decisions about service changes and reconfigurations may be the subject of public consultation but are customarily cast in a form which has only two alternatives – the status quo (by definition unsatisfactory) or the given worked-out proposal. That, in practice, offers only protest or acquiescence as responses: the latter welcomed, the former almost invariably ignored. For how long will that impasse be accepted?

In parallel, on a personal level, choice is an elusive commodity with virtually all the power in the providers' hands. Individual personalised care budgets are in their infancy and regarded with suspicion (will they be guaranteed, realistically inflation proofed?). And given the rigid taxonomy of mental healthcare provision, must the user fit in with the system? The development of co-care with the user (and carer) really sharing the planning of the care pathway and the goal is far from most users' passive reality. The providers of services thus face twin – and perhaps conflicting – pressures, both from commissioners seeking economies and consumers seeking real choices. If choice is to be an everyday reality, it will provoke major changes for users and providers.

ESTABLISHING DESTINATIONS

Curiously, from our riparian viewpoint, as we watch the flow in front of us, we realise that one critical element is absent. While in the acute services targets for reducing mortality and morbidity abound, in the field of mental health only one such goal has been stated. In *Saving Lives*[18] there is only one target:

> to reduce the death rate from suicide and undetermined injury by at least a fifth by 2010.

Progress has been made:

> There were 5906 adult suicides in the UK in 2004, a fall of 7 per cent from the 1991 total of 6366. In 2004 suicides represented 1 per cent of the total of all UK deaths.
>
> This analysis has shown that the strong association between suicide and deprivation shown in previous studies still exists in the 21st century, with rates in deprived areas of England and Wales being double those in the least deprived areas.
>
> **Brock A, Baker A, Griffiths C *et al*. Suicide trends and geographical variations in the UK: 1991–2004. *Health Statistics Quarterly* 2006; 31: 6–22.**

Saving Lives went on to review succinctly but thoroughly the impact and range of mental illness, contributory social factors, the longer-term associated mortality and the economic cost. But as it says:

> . . . we proposed suicide as a proxy target to cover the whole of the mental health priority area. A number of responses to the consultation suggested that a morbidity target would be better but none could offer solutions to the problems of measuring and monitoring such a target.

The *National Service Framework for Mental Health* (*NSF*)[19] has had little to add in terms of outcomes, other than reference to the National Psychiatric Morbidity Survey (a six-yearly monitoring exercise next to be reported on in 2008). This survey may help with some benchmarking but its broad scope is likely to make it difficult to identify cause and effect behind changes in morbidity.

More recently in *Our Health, Our Care, Our Say*,[20] the Department of Health mentions outcomes frequently but without specific references in the field of mental health. Professor Andrew Kerslake looks at outcome-based commissioning and its complexities, saying (with delicate understatement):

> However, there are few practical examples of UK outcome-based contracting on which to draw, and the suspicion is that this may be more difficult to deliver than to describe.[21]

One honourable exception to this picture of random effort has been the hypothesis of applying cognitive behavioural therapy to those unemployed because of ongoing mental illness. This approach (described by Baroness Molly Meacher and Mason Fitzgerald in their chapter in the companion volume *Mental Health Services Today and Tomorrow Part 1: experiences of providing and receiving care*) posits benefits to individuals and society through its application. Some regard it sceptically – and it must be evaluated thoroughly – but it should be measurable and demonstrable in its short- and longer-term effects.

We thus have a picture of a service being reshaped from top to bottom, from hospital to sitting room, with no way at all of discerning whether the changes, investment and upheaval result in improvement to the nation's mental health, or even of significant relief to its quotient of mental illness. One could be forgiven for concluding that this particular social revolution regards mental health services as a likely beneficiary on the basis that if it is thought to improve prisons, social housing and education, it *must* do some good (somehow) for the mentally ill! Obviously lack of evidence does not invalidate the hypothesis but it does make it difficult to comment on very much but process. So there is celebration of the reduction in inpatient admissions due to the spread of community health teams: does that mean faster, more effective, longer-lasting, cheaper (to invoke a few criteria) care? We have a serious gap in our ability to judge success in this new mental health service – and little indication that this picture will change. Are we not interested in defining cure and identifying amelioration?

MAPPING THE DELTA

Having scrutinised and defined the present and the difficulties, we need to look forward and use our present knowledge to suggest what form the flow should take – how can we influence it positively and what should we be trying to achieve? We start by accepting the present as the reality – this is a politically created and politically driven service (you can no more keep politics out of the NHS than you can keep cars off the road!).

There may be modifications to the present shape – some more manoeuvring around the organisational outcrops – but the new philosophy and definitions that we have described are here to stay, whether or not staff and other groups find them congenial. What is not achieved by appealing to hearts and minds can be won via the wallet: did not Aneurin Bevan himself 'stuff mouths with gold'?

Based on our knowledge and researches, we would like to suggest that significant advances could be made by building on present constructs in the following areas: opportunities and rights, clinical inclusion, shaping the service, and balanced and stable investment.

Opportunities and rights

The inter-related social issues that influence and exacerbate mental illness have long been accepted: poverty, unemployment, poor housing and social isolation all contribute (see David McDaid's thorough analysis which follows this chapter). The holistic ideal of intervention would aim to address such factors in the context of an individual's mental illness. But all too often that attention is perfunctory and, with the immediate crisis resolved, the individual's future is left with other agencies. Attempts to draft those agencies into care planning are spasmodic and very mixed in their effectiveness. But if the user were equipped with statutory rights and support, we could expect a more vigorous response from those agencies who would be required to go that step further. Thus the need for a *right* to permanent decent housing and a *right* to employment. The former would be the statutory responsibility of the local authority and the latter that of each employer, who should be required by law to give employment to a number of people professionally diagnosed as suffering from mental illness. Already the Disability Discrimination Act 2005 has strengthened the law with regard to discrimination against individuals because of their mental illness. The expansion of this protection to the requirement actively to employ *and* support individuals with a background of mental illness would be a logical and worthwhile step. The financial, social and emotional benefits of work are well recognised. But all agencies involved would need to support individuals and employers to make this effective.

Our contention is that such legal and statutory emphasis would empower users and carers, oblige agencies to take action and give notice to society of a determination to materially change the status quo.

Clinical inclusion

There is a balance to be found in the context of treatment between the training and experience of professionals and the wishes and motivations of the individual user. It is probably generally accepted that in the 20th century that balance was very tilted towards the professionals. There is pressure to change – but much further to go. The approach to an ideal of shared and informed care, in all but the most extreme situations, should accelerate. Many of the means are there already: the care planning approach, advocacy, the possibility of individual care budgets. But there is an historical reluctance by professionals to share power and acknowledge the individual's contribution to his or her own future. A process-focused service will reduce the individual's worth and institutionalise care, wherever it takes place. Just as care teams are having to adjust in terms of their roles one to another, so a second major adjustment is required in their dealings with users. And not just the tokenism: not the user swamped in the case conference like a living exhibit, but a user supported and made articulate.

In such manner, choice within care and treatment can be made a reality: choice with regard to who, where, when and how. Choice by right not by indulgence; by the financial support of a defined allocation. Thus the user and carer really share in the decision-making: not dominating it, because that, too, would be an imbalance but being able to question and negotiate. And if that is pooh-poohed as too impractical or too complicated, then the very principle of user involvement and individually tailored care is forfeit. This is not visionary theorising; it is the inevitable and welcome outcome of the commitment to customers and choice and should be on every commissioner's and provider's agenda.

Shaping the service

The plural of individual care is public influence. Just as the user and carer should be effective in the specific treatment context, so should the community be in wider considerations affecting services provided and standards achieved. Public confidence will come from awareness and involvement not in a spectator's role watching the team perform, but as contributors to the overall pattern. Public involvement in Foundation Mental Health Trusts needs to be real and significant, not nominal and just numerical. Decisions and choices need to be debated publicly, not simply presented as *faits accomplis*, the apparent 'no brainers' of the present sham of consultation which is almost invariably the presentation of decisions already made. Such a debate and scrutiny will require resources to define and test alternatives.

The process of choosing and reshaping the service should be a public one. This must apply to decisions that providers make and to decisions that commissioners face: both levels should operate in the public interest and in public view. Undoubtedly there will be cries of 'too difficult' and 'commercial – in confidence': these will merely be smokescreens to keep the community at bay because explanation means sharing and sharing means influence.

Future scenarios will include changes and challenges not currently faced (takeovers, amalgamations, new providers and, probably, further national convulsions) but the principle of public involvement in a meaningful way must be maintained.

> Clearly the NHS is going to change dramatically. It will be broken apart and reconstituted into something that more closely resembles a series of 'companies'. Why should anyone now be surprised that this will include joint ventures, mergers and acquisitions?[22]

The community also has a role to play in the context of stigma. Beside the mobilisation of local people to demonstrate the reality of the everyday and understandable experience that most mental illness comprises, the community itself should help to address the fear and anxiety that violence will generate when coupled with mental illnesss. Inquiries into local incidents, including tragedies which have resulted in homicide, serious violence and suicide, could be conducted by a panel including local residents who would be in a better position to represent the community's anxiety and report back to that same community. The need for such inquiries to be more effective is already well established (hundreds of independent inquiries into homicide committed by mentally disordered offenders have broadly made the same recommendations, but apparently with little effect). The model of restorative justice in the criminal justice system has much to offer. Restorative justice allows the parties involved in a specific event to resolve collectively how to deal with the aftermath of that event. A local focus based on past experience, with a properly constituted procedure, which concentrates mainly on systemic faults and inadequacies, could be more effective in terms of learning and communicating. Whatever process is used, it is essential that any changes to the current system of national independent inquiries have the support of the families and secondary victims. The process of inquiries managed locally must be thorough, independent, transparent and in accordance with obligations and responsibilities under human rights legislation.

Balanced and stable investment

In the current climate where an anxious society lacking confidence wants problems locked away, the emphasis has not surprisingly fallen on detention. Provision of secure psychiatric beds has risen sharply and the expenditure on that dramatic minority of patients has doubled in recent years: from £330 million in 2001–02 to £661 million in 2005–06.[23]

No one would wish to return to the institutional inadequacies of the 1970s and 1980s when such provision was lacking or disgraceful, but there is a clear question of the balance of investment. This 'high-risk' care has become the squeaking wheel – amplified by media attention – and has gained increasing attention and significant investment. In the context of a national budget that is unlikely to be able to afford the lavish expansion of the past few years, financial reappraisal is urgently required.

That scrutiny must look at two concurrent issues and establish equity in investment within the NHS budgets. In theory, the new 'market' between commissioners and Foundation Trusts (and other providers) would be described in a series of legally binding contracts which would define costs and service provision, thus establishing a stable budget for mental health services. However, this promised land may be some years away (given the deficiency in commissioning expertise in this area and the gradual promotion of 70-plus Mental Health Trusts to Foundation status). So more immediate action is required.

Firstly it must establish a fixed proportion of the overall budget inalienably committed to mental health services; this should reflect at least the 2005–06 position (that is, if a more sophisticated formula cannot be speedily devised). In other words, 'ring-fenced' allocations to that area of care which cannot be 'raided' to make good deficits in the acute sector. Such an arrangement could be re-examined, say, every five years to see if any evidence was available to change the status quo but a period of stable investment would be guaranteed.

Within that overall limit locally, commissioners would explore competition among providers and, as we have said, involve the communities in that exploration.

Similarly, within that mental health allocation, the investment in forensic facilities should be capped; this may be seen as contentious but there is a danger of unbalanced investment based not so much on clinical priorities as on public anxiety. That cap could be simple – related to last year's expenditure – or it could be more sophisticated, but it needs to be quickly effective.

WATERSHED

The political evolution of the NHS clearly indicates the devices that will be used both to control and to (try to) improve healthcare. These are realities even if they are not yet fully understood or accepted. Part of this movement in mental healthcare has been the flight from the asylum. That phase is virtually complete: now we need to use the flow and current to develop a new mental health service where care is rooted in the community, focused on the individual.

> 'We will treat every patient with dignity and respect.'

> 'We will shape our services around the needs and preferences of individual patients, their families and their carers.'[24]

That individual focus – still only a distant goal in many practical healthcare settings – must be mirrored by a local focus for the change and development in the pattern of care. The long and – in its day – honourable tradition of paternalistic care for passive sufferers is in the past. Active collaboration with informed and supported partners – in individual care or in collective scrutiny – must be the keynote of a new service. Financially secure, mature in its relationship with its communities and with public confidence restored, it should be an outward-looking service ready for change and, above all, responsible to those who fund it.

REFERENCES

 1 Hawe E, editor. *Compendium of Health Statistics: Office of Health Economics.* 18th ed. Oxford: Radcliffe Publishing; 2007.
 2 Hansard. Written Answer; 18 April 2006.
 3 Griffiths R. *NHS Management Inquiry Report.* London: HMSO; 1984.
 4 Cabinet Office. *Policy Review: Public Services.* London: Prime Minister's Strategy Unit; 2007.

5 Ibid.

6 *Health and Personal Social Services Statistics for England.* London: HMSO; 1990.

7 *Health and Personal Social Statistics for England.* London: Department of Health; 2002–03.

8 Personal Communication from Customer Service Centre: Department of Health; 5 March 2007.

9 Prison Reform Trust. Available at: www.prisonreformtrust.org.uk/subsection. asp.12=442

10 Singleton N, Meltzer H, Gatward R, *et al. Psychiatric Morbidity Among Prisoners in England and Wales.* London: HMSO; 1997.

11 Priebe S, Badesconyi A, Fioritti A, *et al.* Reinstitutionalisation in Mental Health Care. *BMJ.* 2005; **330**: 123–6.

12 Scottish Executive. Breaking the mental health taboo. Press release: Scottish Executive; 7 January 2005.

13 Kaye C, Howlett M. *Today and Tomorrow: better services for mental health.* Hay-on-Wye: The Zito Trust; 2005.

14 Rethink. *A Cut Too Far.* London: Rethink; 2006. ('our campaign has so far uncovered over £30 m in cuts in over 30 areas in England'.)

15 Rethink. *A Cut Too Far: six months on.* London: Rethink; 2006. ('a further £37 m of potential cuts'.)

16 Sainsbury Centre for Mental Health. *Under Pressure: the finances of mental health trusts.* London: Sainsbury Centre for Mental Health; 2006.

17 Department of Health. *Community Mental Health Teams. Mental Health Policy Implementation Guide.* London: Department of Health; 2002.

18 Department of Health. *Saving Lives: our healthier nation.* London: Department of Health; 1999.

19 Department of Health. *National Service Framework for Mental Health.* London: Department of Health; 1999.

20 Department of Health. *Our Health, Our Care, Our Say: a new direction for community services.* London: Department of Health; 2006.

21 Kerslake A. *An Approach to Outcome Based Commissioning and Contracting.* London: CSIP; 2006. Available at: www.csip.org.uk

22 Blythe T. Wake up and smell the mergers! *Public Service Magazine.* 2006; September–October.

23 Mental Health Strategies. *National Survey of Investment in Mental Health Services 2005–06.* London: Department of Health; 2006.

24 Department of Health. *NHS Operating Framework.* London: Department of Health; 2005.

CHAPTER 2

The social and economic impact of mental health: meeting the challenge

DAVID McDAID

INTRODUCTION

The consequences of poor mental health are profound. They go way beyond the need for healthcare services. Indeed, what makes poor mental health almost unique is the broad impact it can have on all aspects of life including physical health, family relationships, access to housing and employment, and risk of contact with the criminal justice system. The high levels of public stigma and ignorance associated with mental health problems exacerbate matters, while discrimination increases the likelihood that individuals will become socially excluded.

With so many adverse impacts, it is not surprising to find that the economic costs of poor mental health are also great. Again much of this impact falls not on healthcare services, but is felt elsewhere in the economy, particularly in respect of reduced participation in both paid and unpaid work. These heavy impacts also suggest that interventions effective in preventing or alleviating the consequences of poor mental health have the potential to be highly cost-effective.

This chapter briefly describes some of the principal social and economic impacts of poor mental health that are seen in the United Kingdom (UK), drawing on experience elsewhere in Europe as appropriate. It then considers how these issues may be tackled, illustrating how economic evidence can help by strengthening the case for investment in mental health-related interventions. Other economic incentives can also be used help in deciding how best to co-ordinate actions across different sectors so as to maximise use of available resources to address most efficiently the concerns of those with mental health needs.

WHAT ARE THE CONSEQUENCES OF POOR MENTAL HEALTH?

Health impacts

Mental health problems affect all of us; one in four people experience a significant episode of mental illness during their lifetime, while nearly everyone else will know a family member or friend with mental health problems. The most obvious and stark impact of poor mental health is premature death resulting from suicide. This accounts for 2% of all years of life prematurely lost.[1]

In 2005, 5671 lives were lost as a result of suicide in the UK; while the (three-year rolling) rates per 100 000 of 18.3 for men and 5.9 for women, respectively, are low by European standards and falling, this hides significant geographical differences. For instance, rates of suicide are markedly higher than the national average in Scotland (30.0 for men and 10.0 for women) and Wales (22.4 for men).[2] The rates of suicide in the most deprived areas may be more than double those in the least deprived areas of the UK.[3] The impact does not end with the loss of life; grief and shock can be profound, last many years and have detrimental impacts on the mental health of family and friends. This is to say nothing of the impacts from suicide attempts and deliberate self-harm events.

Poor mental health not only shortens, it also reduces quality of life. The Global Burden of Disease (GBD) is one way of aggregating, for all health problems, all years of life lost prematurely plus all years of life lived in less than full health. According to the GBD, across Europe four of the six leading causes of years lived in less than full health are due to mental health problems: depression, schizophrenia, bipolar disorders and alcohol use disorders.

Only cardiovascular diseases make up a greater share of the GBD, but as illustrated in this chapter, arguably mental health problems have many more consequences across all domains of life. In health terms alone, those living with mental health problems are also more likely to have physical health problems. Evidence from Australia indicates that the risk of developing cardiovascular disease may be four times greater for people with depression compared with the general population.[4]

Employment

Looking beyond narrow health impacts, in both the UK and elsewhere in Europe, those with long-standing mental health problems are far less likely to be employed than the general working-age population.[5,6] The majority of European countries with data report employment rates of around 20–30%. There are limited data by diagnosis but employment rates for people with psychotic disorders are usually lower than those for other long-term mental health problems. Recent research in England also suggests that individuals with mental health problems have up to a 40% lower chance of obtaining employment compared with other disability groups.[7]

While it is difficult to make direct comparisons, there do appear to be substantial variations across Europe. Italy, for instance, reports employment rates of 46.5% for all diagnoses compared with 18.4% in the UK.[8] Emerging research suggests that these differences may be a product of different socio-economic contexts, including the structure of disability benefit systems.[9–11] In part, this is also due to discrimination encountered within the labour market. Others contend that there may be an element of self-discrimination, too, by people with mental health difficulties who may believe that they have no chance of obtaining employment.[12] In addition, mental health professionals have been charged with discouraging individuals from seeking work, for fear that this will be ultimately be unsuccessful and lead to undue hardship if disability benefits are difficult to regain.[13]

Although the focus here is on reduced opportunities to enter into employment as part of the recovery process, it should be noted that mental health problems can also be triggered by the working environment. Across the European Union (EU) there is evidence of a trend of increasing absenteeism and early retirement due to mental health problems; in many instances poor mental health is the principal reason for sickness absence.[14] In the Netherlands between 1970 and 2003, for example, there was a steady increase in the risk of workers being registered as disabled because of a psychological disorder; by 2003 they accounted for 35% of all new disability claimants.[15]

Housing and criminal justice

The lack of fair opportunities for people with mental health problems, poor recognition of mental health needs by professionals in different sectors and/or a lack of appropriate support services can also contribute to other adverse impacts. Individuals can have a much higher chance of becoming homeless than the general population; this does not simply mean having no roof but also includes those living in a range of far-from-ideal temporary accommodation.

A lack of financial security can also make it more difficult to remain in the private rented sector or to obtain long-term accommodation.[16] One English survey of more than 1500 people living rough or in hostels reported that more than 40% had mental health problems,[17] while the Psychiatric Morbidity Survey for Great Britain found that almost half of all people with mental health problems were in local authority or housing association accommodation compared with 15% of those without mental health problems.[18]

Individuals with mental health problems are also more likely to come into contact with the criminal justice system; indeed, it has been estimated that as many as 90% of the prison population in Great Britain have a mental health disorder (although many mental health problems, such as depression and anxiety, arise within prison). In some instances, however, individuals may be sent to prison because of the lack of opportunity for treatment and support in a non-custodial environment.[19]

Long-term impacts from childhood to adulthood

One area which has received much attention in recent years has been the long-term adverse impacts on children of mental health problems. Although data are limited, there are several long-term studies in the UK and elsewhere which report that, compared to 'normal' children, those who had childhood mental health problems appear in adulthood to have much higher rates of contact with the criminal justice system in particular, poorer family relationships and less stable employment. When working, there is a tendency to earn less, although the evidence here is mixed.[20–23]

Consequences for families

Poor mental health can have a substantial impact on families. There can be worry and concern over the health and long-term future of a loved one.[24] There may be concerns about behaviour such as restlessness, hypochondria, sleep disturbances or aggressiveness.[25] In many cases, family members may find that they have to devote considerable time every day to providing support and informal care to a loved one. This may reduce their own opportunities to maintain employment and social activities. Partners of people with persistent depression report marked difficulties in maintaining social and leisure activities, complain about a decrease in total family income, and may have considerable strains placed on their marital relationships.[26,27]

There can also be long-term impacts on the children of people with mental health problems. They may suffer from neglect and, although few hard data are available, older children may sometimes find themselves providing much care and support.[28] As a consequence, schooling may be disrupted, potentially curtailing long-term opportunities in adulthood.

ECONOMIC IMPACT

Each of these personal and social impacts is associated with enormous economic costs. Global estimates vary, but very conservatively the costs of common depression and anxiety-related disorders, in addition to those for psychotic disorders, have been estimated to account for at least 4% of a country's annual economic output.[29] Some UK estimates, that more unusually also place a monetary value on the grief and distress associated with poor mental health, have suggested that the costs of all mental health problems may be as high as 9% of UK economic output.[30] All cost estimates are, however, just that – estimates – and need to be treated with great caution; methods used in their calculation can vary significantly, so meaningful comparisons are far from straightforward. Some aspects of cost are outlined below.

Lost productivity

In contrast to the costs associated with many physical health problems, the majority of quantified costs associated with mental health problems occur outside the health and social care sector. Most studies have not sought to put a value on the grief and distress associated with poor mental health, so the majority of costs usually are due to lost opportunities for employment, as well as absenteeism, poor performance within the workplace and premature retirement. Typically these lost productivity costs account for between 60% and 80% of the total economic impact of major mental health problems.[31] Analysis of data from the UK Quarterly Labour Force Survey also indicates that employees with mental health problems may be absent around five times more often than those with other health problems.[32]

The impacts of mental health on employment have knock-on implications in terms of hiring and training costs, reduced potential for economic growth, lost taxation revenue and higher social security payments. Indeed, the sustainability of social protection systems may be challenged by substantial increases in disability benefits paid to those people who have left work on grounds of poor mental health. In the UK, incapacity benefits paid to people with mental health problems far outweigh all payments for unemployment benefit.

Looking at depression alone, it has been estimated that the cost to the English economy was £9.055 billion in 2002. The impact on national productivity in terms of absenteeism, premature retirement from the labour force and suicide (thus losing the opportunity to be productive) expressed in cost terms was 23 times larger than the costs falling to the health service.[33] Another more recent estimate put the cost to the economy of depression and anxiety-related disorders at £17 billion.[34]

These are not isolated findings: millions of working days are lost each year throughout Europe because of depression-related disorders, e.g. 31.9 million lost working days in France in 2000 were attributed to depression.[35] In total across Europe, the costs of depression were estimated to be €118 billion in 2004, of which €76 billion was due to productivity losses from poor health and premature mortality.[36] Although in absolute terms their numbers are much smaller, people living with psychotic disorders such as schizophrenia still have substantial non-health system costs. Many European studies, such as those in England and Hungary, report that health and social care costs account for just one-third of all costs, with the other two-thirds being due to lost employment.[37]

Despite this, the productivity-related impact of cost has often remained 'hidden'; if anything, the findings are also conservative. They typically do not include losses of productivity from unpaid activities, such as a reduction in the ability to care for one's children or partake in voluntary work. From an economic perspective, these should be seen as part of the total costs of poor mental health. Moreover, the costs of reduced performance at work by people with untreated mental health problems may be five times as great as those for absenteeism, but only limited research has examined this issue.[38]

This would suggest that it is not enough to simply help individuals return to employment; a commitment is also required to ongoing measures to reduce this risk of drop-out from work and also more generally to foster mental well-being in the workplace. Even if the potential productive capacity of some people with mental health problems may be less than that in the general population, the majority are capable of work and wish to engage in it. The magnitude of potential costs that might be avoided through effective interventions should provide a powerful incentive to those funding welfare benefit systems to invest in employment-related measures as a mechanism on the path to recovery.

Suicide

Most suicides are related to mental health problems and incur substantial costs. These include not only emergency services, potential life-saving healthcare interventions, police and coroner investigations and funerals, but again the lost lifetime opportunity to contribute productively to the national economy, whether this be through paid work, voluntary activities or family responsibilities. In addition, there is the loss of the opportunity to experience all that life holds. The pain and grief that suicide can inflict on immediate family members and friends can be immense. While it might intuitively seem strange to place a monetary value on these intangible factors, these costs are routinely included by policy-makers in some other sectors – most notably in transport, when looking at the case for investing in measures to reduce the risk of transport-related deaths. Clearly for policy-makers to make a fully informed choice, say, between new car safety measures and measures to reduce the chances to suicide, it is important to consider costs on a level playing field.

Using this comprehensive approach, the lifetime costs of all suicides in Scotland in 2004 were recently estimated to be almost £1.08 billion with 75% due to suicides by men.[39] This represents an average cost of £1.29 million per completed suicide and is comparable to estimates reported in New Zealand and Ireland.[40,41] By far the largest single component of the total costs of suicide (more than 70%) is that of the intangible human costs experienced by families; in addition, lost productivity costs account for a further 21% of total costs.

Long-term costs for children

The broad nature of the costs of poor mental health can also be seen in long-term studies of children. In one study of children with persistent antisocial behaviour in London, only 5% of the total cost was carried by the health service, with the remainder falling to schools (special educational needs), social care agencies, community voluntary organisations, families (disrupted parental employment, household damage) and the welfare system (disability and similar transfer payments).[42] Another London-based study that followed children, identified at age 10 as having conduct disorder, generated by age 27 costs for a range of agencies that were significantly higher than the costs for a non-morbid control group (£70 000 versus £7500); most noticeable were the criminal justice system costs, which were 18 times greater.[43]

Cost to families

It is tempting for policy-makers to view the desire and willingness of family members to provide care and support as a 'free' resource. However, it can entail significant economic costs for individuals and society. Family carers give up time which they otherwise could have used for work or leisure. They may also incur additional out-of-pocket expenses to support a relative financially and require treatment for their own physical and mental health problems.

Remarkably little UK data is available, but one Italian study (albeit that Italy is a country where traditionally the family has a greater input) estimated that 20% of the costs associated with schizophrenia were due to lost employment, employment opportunities foregone and the leisure-time costs of family carers.[44] In Australia, the annual costs for 2379 carers of people with schizophrenia who had to give up the opportunity to work ranged from $AUS 51.5 million[45] to $AUS 88 million, or just over 6% of the total cost.[46] The authors of this latter study considered this estimate to be conservative as it did not include the costs for part-time carers or those not designated as 'home carers'.

THE WAY FORWARD

The personal, social and economic impacts of mental illness are profound. Costs alone are, however, an insufficient reason for investing in measures to improve mental health – such investment can only be considered if effective actions that might help to reduce the adverse socio-economic impacts of poor mental health are taken as well. It is also important to consider whether this is an appropriate use of what will always be a finite level of resources.

The good news is that the case for action (for many areas of poor mental health) appears well justified in terms of the availability of effective clinical interventions. Intuitively the economic benefits of reducing the long-term consequences of poor mental health through a broad range of interventions that not only deal with clinical symptoms but also promote social inclusion and help, and which empower individuals to achieve their potential in education, work and family life appear increasingly attractive, but the evidence base is still weak.

Using economics to strengthen the case for investment

Economic evidence can be used to help facilitate change. One key issue is to make the case for greater investment even more compelling by continuing to build and strengthen the evidence base on the cost-effectiveness of not only medical treatments for mental health disorders where the evidence base is quite robust,[47-52] but also of those more holistic interventions that may help to reduce social exclusion and promote independent living. For instance, while there are some encouraging but often US-based studies suggesting that interventions are cost-effective, more information is needed on the potential long-term benefits of early interventions in school and on interventions to help individuals obtain employment on the open labour market (see later in section).

Is the obvious next step to invest more resources in cost-effective interventions for mental health? Unfortunately it is not that simple. While additional resources are always welcome, compared with the situation in most other countries in Europe mental health in the UK already appears to receive a reasonable share of the healthcare budget (around 13% in England).[53] In addition to investing in proven effective interventions, there is a need for improved co-ordination and co-operation across sectors.[54] Investment in actions to help individuals return to work in particular seems merited; this, however, will require more than public resources – it will also need support from both employers and fellow employees.

Moving towards a more seamless provision of services that meet needs

One key challenge is the fragmented nature of the support system; interventions inevitably must be provided across a number of sectors, including employment, housing and education. From the service user perspective the aim should be to provide a 'seamless' service package regardless of the source of funding or affiliation of the service provider.

One way of facilitating a more joined-up approach may be through the greater use of joint budgets between health, social care and other sectors, as appropriate. While evaluation of experience with such pooled budgets for mental health-specific services remains limited, experience in other areas is encouraging. In Sweden, for example, experiments in pooling budgets between Health, Social Services and the sickness insurance budget have, in part, been set up to respond to the growing problem of long-term absence from the labour market because of mental health problems.[55] Up to 5% of Social Services and sickness insurance budgets can be pooled together with a matching contribution from Health services. Initial analysis across eight county councils, in respect of people with musculo-skeletal problems, suggests that interdisciplinary co-ordination and collaboration has improved.

Economic incentives and/or disincentives might also be used to help encourage a more appropriate use of resources. In England, since 2003, local Social Services can be penalised by £100 per day (£120 in London) for each older person whose discharge from hospital is delayed by more than three days. Delays have reduced but the merits of extending this scheme to mental health service users are mixed.[56] While it might help in shifting resources, there are concerns that introducing a 'blame culture' might harm developing partnership arrangements between healthcare and social care services. Similarly, concerns exist that so-called 'trans-institutionalisation' might occur with individuals placed in inappropriate social service-funded care facilities, rather than in the community, in order to avoid these financial penalties.

Making use of financial arrangements to empower service users

A better approach might be to link available funds directly to individual service users, for instance through the use of direct payments. These cash payments can empower individuals to plan for and purchase services that best meet their needs, regardless of sector; thus such payments are also consistent with initiatives to promote greater individual choice and might overcome some of the challenges of a fragmented delivery system. It might also mean that more funding could become available for less traditional services, such as job coaching within supported employment schemes, or education and training courses.

Little evaluation of direct payments for people with mental health needs has as yet been undertaken and uptake to date is very limited. In England by March 2005 this represented just 0.6% of the total mental health service client group and just 4% of all those receiving direct payments.[57,58] Similar figures have been reported in Scotland.[59] One study of 60 English mental health service users did show that about half used funds to pay for personal assistants, while others used the money to pay for items such as transport, education and leisure activities.[60]

Actions to help support individuals who wish to obtain/return to employment

Potentially, given that productivity losses are responsible for much of the costs of poor mental health, interventions that can help individuals to return to work or prevent mental health problems occurring in the workplace may be highly cost-effective. The weight of evidence on the effectiveness of one approach to supported employment – where individuals are placed in open employment and then receive ongoing support, known as individual placement and support (IPS) – compared with vocational rehabilitation, is strong. Moreover, what evidence is available, although largely from the US, suggests that economic productivity is enhanced more by IPS schemes, measured in terms of more hours of work and higher wage rates, than by traditional vocational rehabilitation schemes.[61,62]

In one review, Latimer reports that converting day treatment or other less effective vocational programmes to supported employment can be cost-saving or cost-neutral, from the hospital, community centre and government points of view.[63] He has also suggested that the success of the IPS model may be generalisable to the very different context to be found outside the US.[64] A six-country (including England) European Commission-supported study, EQOLISE, has recently investigated the cost-effectiveness of supported employment for people with severe mental illness, using the IPS model compared with existing vocational services. Results from this study should be in the public domain soon and may potentially provide much impetus for more investment (*see* www.eqolise.sgul.ac.uk/ for more information). The Pathways to Work initiative in England, which involves a pro-active programme of support and advice to those on long-term disability benefits, on how to return to work, training to enhance skills, as well as support while at work, is also the subject of ongoing evaluation.[65]

Of course, stable employment is just one outcome of IPS. In comparison with other employment-related interventions, higher rates of employment can be associated with other benefits such as reduced need for healthcare services, increased levels of social inclusion and improved quality of life. Even if individuals still move in and out of employment after receiving supported employment, their use of health and other support services may be reduced considerably during times of employment. One 11-year US evaluation following 3000 employment service clients for 48 months, reported that overall costs were lower because the use of health services was much lower during periods of stable employment.[66]

It would be erroneous for the reader to draw the conclusion that this discussion represents a comprehensive view of ways to encourage open employment. There are many other interventions, some of which would merit more detailed discussion. One area, for instance, where further work is needed is in respect of the use of cognitive training programmes as an element of supported employment – these may be particularly targeted at those for whom employment does not seem to last. This may complement work done using cognitive approaches to tackle problems for people already in the workforce.[34] Contextual factors will also have a bearing on the success with which individuals with mental health difficulties obtain open employment; these factors relate to employment law, as well as to equal opportunities and diversity policies.

Welfare reform

It needs to be recognised that the success of interventions may be very dependent on benefit systems; for instance, some in a European context have argued that disability benefits can inappropriately act as a disincentive to return to work. For instance, if an individual obtains employment but then loses his or her job, it may take a considerable period of time to reclaim disability benefits, during which time significant hardship may be endured.[67] Ensuring that there are financial benefits from a return to work is also important. As part of the Pathways to Work programme, a system of tax credits and additional return-to-work credits – paid as a supplement to earnings during the first year of work – has been introduced. Recent qualitative analysis suggests that this financial support, if effective, is of key importance in getting people back to work; when payments are delayed or not claimed, financial problems occur quickly.[68]

CONCLUSION

In summary, poor mental health is a major public health issue in the UK and elsewhere in Europe; it has many health and socio-economic consequences for individuals and their families, as well as for society generally. There is undoubtedly a greater recognition of the importance of mental health in Europe, as evidenced by the intergovernmental conference on mental health in Helsinki in January 2005, under the auspices of the World Health Organization, European Union, Council of Europe and the Government of Finland. The need to tackle the economic impacts of poor mental health was one critical element of the declaration and action plan endorsed in Helsinki.[69]

The view is that greater investment in many areas of mental health is not only justified on grounds of tackling the high degree of social exclusion and adverse health consequences, but that it also represents a more efficient use of health (and other sector) resources, allowing many individuals to maintain or regain their normal role, making an active contribution to society either through paid or unpaid work. There are of course areas where careful evaluation in a UK and/or European context is still required to plug gaps in our knowledge; different mechanisms to help individuals to obtain employment as part of the path to recovery are one particular case in point.

Exploiting these potential benefits will require more than greater investment in cost-effective interventions. This should not be equated with demonstrating that interventions save money, but rather that greater investment leads to improved personal and social-economic outcomes. It also necessitates arguing for organisational and structural reforms to help ensure that interventions best meet the needs of mental health service users, regardless of whether they are delivered within the health, social care, education, employment, housing or criminal justice sectors.

REFERENCES

1 World Health Organization. *Suicide prevention website.* Geneva: World Health Organization; 2005. Available at: www.who.int/mental_health/prevention/suicide/suicideprevent/en
2 Office of National Statistics. *Suicide data 1991–2004.* London: Office of National Statistics; 2007.
3 Brock A, Baker A, Griffiths C, *et al.* Suicide trends and geographical variations in the United Kingdom, 1991–2004. *Health Stat Q.* 2006; **31**: 6–22.
4 Lawrence D, Holman CDJ, Jablensky AV. *Preventable Physical Illness in People with Mental Illness.* Perth: University of Western Australia; 2001.
5 Smith A, Twomey B. Labour market experiences of people with disabilities. *Labour Market Trends* 2002; **August**: 415–27.

6 Marwaha S, Johnson S. Schizophrenia and employment: a review. *Soc Psychiatry Psychiatr Epidemiol.* 2004; **39**: 337–49.

7 Berthoud R. *The Employment Rates of Disabled People.* London: Department of Work and Pensions; 2006.

8 Curran C, Knapp M, McDaid D, *et al.* Mental health and employment: an overview of patterns and policies across the 17 MHEEN countries. *J Ment Health.* 2007; **16**(2): 195–210.

9 Drake RE, Fox T, Leather P, *et al.* Regional variation in competitive employment for persons with severe mental illness. *Adm Policy Ment Health.* 1998; **25**(5): 493–504.

10 Becker DR, Xie H, McHugo GJ, *et al.* What predicts supported employment program outcomes? *Community Ment Health J.* 2006; **42**(3): 303–13.

11 Kilian R, Becker T. Macro-economic indicators and labour force participation of people with schizophrenia. *J Ment Health.* 2007;**16**(2): 211–22.

12 Thornicroft G. *Actions Speak Louder . . . tackling discrimination against people with mental illness.* London: Mental Health Foundation; 2006.

13 Office of the Deputy Prime Minister. *Mental Health and Social Exclusion.* Social Exclusion Unit report. London: Office of the Deputy Prime Minister; 2004.

14 Wynne R, MacAnaney D. *Employment and Disability: back to work strategies.* Dublin: European Foundation for the Improvement of Living and Working Conditions; 2004.

15 Statistics Netherlands. *Statistics Netherlands website.* 2004. Available at: www.cbs.nl/en-GB/default.htm

16 Anderson R, Wynne R, McDaid D. Housing and employment. In: Knapp M, McDaid D, Mossialos E, *et al*, editors. *Mental Health Policy and Practice Across Europe.* Buckingham: Open University Press, McGraw-Hill; 2006: 280–307.

17 St Mungo's. *St Mungo's Big Survey into the Problems and Lives of Homeless People.* London: St Mungo's; 2004.

18 Meltzer H, Singleton N, Lee A, *et al. The Social and Economic Circumstances of Adults with Mental Disorders.* London: HMSO; 2002.

19 All Party Parliamentary Group on Prison Health. *The Mental Health Problem in UK HM Prisons.* London: House of Commons; 2006.

20 Scott S, Knapp M, Henderson J, *et al.* Financial cost of social exclusion: follow up study of antisocial children into adulthood. *BMJ.* 2001; **323**: 191–6.

21 Chen H, Cohen P, Kasen S, *et al.* Impact of adolescent mental disorders and physical illnesses on quality of life 17 years later. *Arch Pediatr Adolesc Med.* 2006; **160**(1): 93–9.

22 Knapp M, McCrone P, Fombonne E, *et al.* The Maudsley long term follow up of child and adolescent depression. *Br J Psych.* 2002; **180**: 19–23.

23 McCrone P, Knapp M, Fombonne E. The Maudsley long-term follow-up of child and adolescent depression. Predicting costs in adulthood. *Eur Child Adolesc Psychiatry.* 2005; **14**(7): 407–13.

24 Thornicroft G, Tansella M, Becker T, *et al.* The personal impact of schizophrenia in Europe. *Schizophr Res.* 2004; **69**(2–3): 125–32.

25 Schene AH, van Wijngaarden B, Koeter MW. Family caregiving in schizophrenia: domains and distress. *Schizophr Bull.* 1998; **24**(4): 609–18.

26 van Wijngaarden B, Schene AH, Koeter MW. Family caregiving in depression: impact on caregivers' daily life, distress, and help seeking. *J Affect Disord.* 2004; **81**(3): 211–22.

27 Jungbauer J, Wittmund B, Dietrich S, *et al*. The disregarded caregivers: subjective burden in spouses of schizophrenia patients. *Schizophr Bull*. 2004; **30**(3): 665–75.

28 Ostman M, Hansson L. Children in families with a severely mentally ill member. Prevalence and needs for support. *Soc Psychiatry Psychiatr Epidemiol*. 2002; **37**: 243–8.

29 Gabriel P, Liimatainen M-R. *Mental Health in the Workplace*. Geneva: International Labour Organisation; 2000.

30 Sainsbury Centre for Mental Health. *Economic and Social Costs of Mental Illness in England*. London: Sainsbury Centre for Mental Health; 2003.

31 McDaid D, Curran C, Knapp M. Promoting mental well-being in the workplace: a European policy perspective. *Int Rev Psychiatry* 2005; **17**(5): 365–73.

32 Almond S, Healey A. Mental health and absence from work: new evidence from the UK Quarterly Labour Force Survey. *Work, Employment and Society*. 2003; **17**(4): 731–42.

33 Thomas C, Morris S. Cost of depression among adults in England in 2000. *Br J Psych*. 2003; **183**: 514–19.

34 Layard R. The case for psychological treatment centres. *BMJ*. 2006; **332**: 1030–2.

35 Bejean S, Sultan-Taieb H. Modelling the economic burden of diseases imputable to stress at work. *Eur J Health Econ*. 2005; **50**: 16–23.

36 Sobocki P, Jonsson B, Angst J, *et al*. Cost of depression in Europe. *J Ment Health Policy Econ*. 2006; **9**(2): 87–98.

37 Knapp M, Mangalore R, Simon J. The global costs of schizophrenia. *Schizophr Bull*. 2004; **2**: 297–303.

38 Kessler RC, Frank RG. The impact of psychiatric disorders on work loss days. *Psychol Med*. 1997; **27**: 861–73.

39 Platt S, Halliday E, Maxwell M, *et al*. *Evaluation of the first phase of Choose Life. Final Report*. Edinburgh: Scottish Executive; 2006.

40 Kennelly B, Ennis J, O'Shea E. The economic cost of suicide and deliberate self harm in Ireland. In: *'Reach Out' a National Strategy for Action on Suicide Prevention*. Dublin: Department of Health and Children; 2005.

41 O'Dea D, Tucker S. *The Cost of Suicide to Society*. Wellington: New Zealand Ministry of Health; 2005.

42 Romeo R, Knapp M, Scott S. Economic cost of severe antisocial behaviour in children – and who pays for it? *Br J Psych*. 2006; **188**: 547–53.

43 Scott S, Knapp M, Henderson J, *et al*. Op. cit.

44 Tarricone R, Gerzeli S, Montanelli, R *et al*. Direct and indirect costs of schizophrenia in community psychiatric services in Italy. The GISIES study. Interdisciplinary Study Group on the Economic Impact of Schizophrenia. *Health Pol*. 2000; **51**(1): 1–18.

45 Carr VJ, Neil AL, Halpin SA, *et al*. Costs of schizophrenia and other psychoses in urban Australia: findings from the Low Prevalence (Psychotic) Disorders Study. *Aust NZ J Psych*. 2003; **37**: 31–40.

46 Access Economics. *Schizophrenia: costs. An analysis of the burden of schizophrenia and related suicide in Australia*. Melbourne: SANE Australia; 2002.

47 Barrett B, Byford S, Knapp M. Evidence of cost-effective treatments for depression: a systematic review. *J Affect Disord*. 2005; **84**(1): 1–13.

48 Chisholm D, Sanderson K, Ayuso-Mateos JL, *et al*. Reducing the global burden of depression: population-level analysis of intervention cost-effectiveness in 14 world regions. *Br J Psych*. 2004; **184**: 393–403.

49 Knapp M, Barrett B, Romeo R, *et al. An International Review of Cost-Effectiveness Studies for Mental Disorders*. Washington, DC: Fogarty International Center of the National Institutes of Health; 2004. Working Paper 36.

50 Lothgren M. Economic evidence in psychotic disorders: a review. *Eur J Health Econ.* 2004; 5(Suppl 1): S67–74.

51 Lothgren M. Economic evidence in anxiety disorders: a review. *Eur J Health Econ* 2004; 5(Suppl 1): S20–5.

52 Romeo R, Byford S, Knapp M. Economic evaluations of child and adolescent mental health interventions: a systematic review. *J Child Psychol Psychiatry.* 2005; 46: 919–30.

53 Knapp M, McDaid D, Ammadeo F, *et al.* Financing mental health care in Europe. *J Ment Health.* 2007; 16(2): 167–80.

54 McDaid D, Oliveira MD, Jurczak K, *et al.* Moving beyond the mental health care system: an exploration of the interfaces between health and non-health sectors. *J Ment Health.* 2007; 16(2): 181–94.

55 Hultberg EL, Glendinning C, Allebeck P, *et al.* Using pooled budgets to integrate health and welfare services: a comparison of experiments in England and Sweden. *Health Soc Care Community.* 2005; 13(6): 531–41.

56 Lewis R, Glasby J. Delayed discharge from mental health hospitals: results of an English postal survey. *Health Soc Care Community.* 2006; 14(3): 225–30.

57 Davey V, Fernandez J-L, Knapp M, *et al. Direct Payments Survey: a national survey of direct payments policy and practice.* London: Personal Social Services Research Unit; 2006.

58 Information Centre. *Personal Social Services expenditure and unit costs: England: 2004–2005.* Available at: www.ic.nhs.uk/pubs/persocservexp2005

59 Direct Payments Scotland. *Direct Payments for Users of Mental Health Services.* Dundee pilot report. Edinburgh: Direct Payments Scotland; 2005.

60 Spandler H, Vick N. Opportunities for independent living using direct payments in mental health. *Health Soc Care Community.* 2006; 14(2): 107–15.

61 Cook JA, Leff HS, Blyler CR, *et al.* Results of a multisite randomized trial of supported employment interventions for individuals with severe mental illness. *Arch Gen Psychiatry.* 2005; 62(5): 505–12.

62 Crowther R, Marshall M, Bond G, *et al.* Vocational rehabilitation for people with severe mental illness. *Cochrane Database Syst Rev.* 2001; 2: CD003080.

63 Latimer EA. Economic impacts of supported employment for persons with severe mental illness. *Can J Psychiatry.* 2001; 46(6): 496–505.

64 Latimer EA, Lecomte T, Becker DR, *et al.* Generalisability of the individual placement and support model of supported employment: results of a Canadian randomised controlled trial. *Br J Psychiatry.* 2006; 189: 65–73.

65 Blyth B. *Incapacity Benefit Reforms: Pathways to Work pilots performance and analysis.* London: Department of Work and Pensions. Working Paper 26; 2006.

66 Perkins DV, Born DL, Raines JA, *et al.* Program evaluation from an ecological perspective: supported employment services for persons with serious psychiatric disabilities. *Psychiatr Rehabil J.* 2005; 28(3): 217–24.

67 Organisation for Economic Co-operation and Development. *Transforming Disability into Ability: policies to promote work and income security for disabled people.* Paris: OECD; 2003.

68 Corden A, Nice K. *Incapacity Benefit Reforms Pilot: findings from the second cohort in a longitudinal panel of clients.* Research Report 345. London: Department of Work and Pensions; 2006.

69 World Health Organization. *Mental Health Declaration for Europe: facing the challenges, building solutions.* Copenhagen: World Health Organization; 2005.

CHAPTER 3

Central control and local freedom: a new balance

ALAN MAYNARD

INTRODUCTION

There is continual debate about the balance between local freedom to deliver mental health services and central control of standards and performance, with much talk about increasing local autonomy and much policy action that centralises finance and care for patients. The essence of the National Health Service (NHS) is providing access to healthcare on the basis of need. Of course, this concept has to be defined with care. Is need to be defined from the perspective of the individual patient? – that is, I feel ill and should be cared for regardless of whether you, as a healthcare provider, can improve my mental and physical well-being? Or is it to be defined from the perspective of the evidence base about the clinical and cost-effectiveness of interventions available to treat presenting patients?

The assumption generally used in the NHS is the latter, i.e. need exists when there is an intervention available to treat the patient in a clinically effective way, and access to needed or clinically effective care will be made available in relation to the relative cost-effectiveness of competing clinically effective treatments.[1,2] This perspective increasingly dominates resource allocation advice through regulatory mechanisms such as the National Institute for Health and Clinical Excellence (NICE). The desire to achieve equity in access to cost-effective healthcare has led to the use of regulatory mechanisms that inevitably centralise control.

The argument in this chapter is that because of this egalitarian goal and related factors, which will be discussed subsequently, local freedom to vary service delivery will always be highly constrained. In a national health service, the policy focus must always be on treating need regardless of willingness and ability to pay. This requires firstly, the identification of 'what works' cost-effectively and secondly, creating incentives to ensure that what is cost-effective is delivered to patients in need.

Failure to identify what works cost-effectively and to incentivise its delivery is commonplace in many public and private healthcare systems.[3] This is often the product of local discretion, sometimes disguised as 'clinical autonomy', where providers may ignore the evidence base and experiment unethically on their patients outside properly constructed and implemented clinical trials. The exercise of such autonomy, when inefficient, is unethical as it deprives potential patients of care from which they could benefit.

The challenge of designing and implementing efficient national rationing mechanisms is the subject of the next section and is followed by discussion of giving incentives for the translation into practice of evidence of cost-effectiveness.

RATIONING HEALTHCARE: THE INEVITABLE AND THE UBIQUITOUS

Whether mentally or physically ill – and increasingly the two domains overlap considerably – the patient faces a variety of rationing devices in all sectors of the healthcare system. The individual's decision to consult may be constrained or augmented by family members and their capacity to tend the unwell in informal care settings. Once in the formal healthcare system, the patient may find that a doctor or nurse becomes their principal agent, determining what services and support are given. However, often in mental ill-health, the family carer, spouse or partner may continue to play a central role in ensuring, for instance, medication compliance, psychological support and behaviour moderation. Rationing is conducted by the patient, the family and many actors in the public and private parts of the health system.

Rationing involves depriving the patient of care from which they could benefit and which they wish to consume. Thus for the drug addict or the alcoholic, the family may try to moderate behaviour and assist recovery. Their need for help may result in their approaching the primary care system. This system is often quite poor at delivering care, for instance because of failure to diagnose depression. The addict might also use statutory support in the hospital or be cared for by a private sector drug treatment agency. Typically the patient's pathway is fragmented and the service consumption is disrupted by lapses in patient perseverance and service integration.

However, fragmentation in care is a product not only of the jigsaw nature of public and private provision, but also of lack of evidence about the clinical and cost-effectiveness of many interventions in healthcare. Skrabanek and McCormick, both physicians, have pleaded for the spreading of 'scepticaemia' about medicine. They define 'scepticaemia' as 'an uncommon generalised disorder of low infectivity. Medical school education is likely to confer lifelong immunity.'[4]

The evidence base about what works or is clinically effective in medicine is incomplete. A recent 'guestimate' concluded that over 45% of the physician's armoury had no evidence base. This is not to say it is useless, but neither is it appropriate to say it works. We simply are uncertain about a considerable number of healthcare interventions[5] and have to recognise that these continue to be used by practitioners.

This uncertainty about the effectiveness of care given to patients should drive investment in clinical trials. Sadly the funding of independent research remains relatively poor and trials are generally driven by industry. Pharmaceutical companies have to show that new products are safe, efficacious and of quality. After testing on animals, companies evaluate the effects of new products on humans. However, these trials may meet regulatory requirements and yet be unsatisfactory in terms of demonstrating clinical effectiveness, let alone informing the modelling of cost-effectiveness.

The first weakness that can be detected in clinical trails is the choice of comparator. If you invent the potential wonder drug X, there is a nice issue of what you compare it with in a trial. Should it be the most commonly used alternative or the cheapest alternative? The regulations continue to permit comparison with a placebo, which enables us to detect effect but not comparative effect.

A nice example of practice with regard to choice of comparator is a study of a new drug for the treatment of schizophrenia, in which an optimal dose of the new chemical entity was compared with the established treatment at a level several times greater than the recommended dose.[6] Unsurprisingly the side-effects profile of the older drug showed it was 'inferior' to the new one. This sort of 'analysis' when published, as it often is due to poor peer review, is used for marketing to practitioners.

Another problem inherent in many trials is their duration. With industry claiming that successful drugs cost about $800 million to bring to market, companies are anxious to get product licences and market their innovation as soon as possible. As a consequence, they favour short trials. This has well-recognised problems, epitomised by Vioxx, a Cox2 inhibitor used to control acute pain in arthritis. This product got a licence after short-term trial results demonstrated its efficacy. However, the results after 12–18 months showed significantly increased risk of adverse cardiac effects and the drug had to be taken off the market.[7]

Chalmers has emphasised how there needs to be more evaluation of biological research to demonstrate that we get value for money. As he shows, most biological research funding is used in basic science for 'underpinning' and 'aetiological' investigations whose pay-offs are unclear and may be long term. Only 10% of biological research goes into the evaluation of treatments.[8] He concludes that 'poor basic research has resulted in treatments either useless or harmful'.

His strictures about the proper use of scientific rigour in the design, execution and reporting of trials lead him to three provocative but insightful conclusions:[9]

1 'because professionals sometimes do more harm than good when they intervene in the lives of other people, their policies and practices should be informed by rigorous, transparent, up to date evaluations' (at page 24)
2 'surveys often reveal wide variations in the type and frequency of practice and policy interventions, and this evidence of collective uncertainty should prompt humility that is a precondition for rigorous evaluation' (at page 27)
3 'evaluation should begin with systematic assessment of as high a proportion as possible of existing, relevant research, and then, if appropriate, additional research' (at page 30)

The biases in the evidence base created by poor scientific method are a considerable problem for those seeking to identify what works. The pharmaceutical industry is driven by profit and, at the margin, some of its marketing techniques are clearly not helpful to those concerned with the efficient deployment of scarce healthcare resources. These problems have been well chronicled and involve selective use of evidence in marketing, non-revelation of data that fail to generate profit, and inappropriate relations with practitioners.[10,11]

Improving the quality and quantity of research into clinical effectiveness and its transparency are preconditions for improving evidence about the cost-effectiveness of competing interventions used to treat patients. Such information is essential for prioritising competing claims for funding and is now central to the work of NICE (www.nice.org.uk).

NICE evaluates health technologies and produces clinical guidelines, and more recently has been given the role of identifying the evidence base for health promotion and illness prevention interventions. Its agenda is determined by

Ministers and its guidance is mandatory, meaning that if clinicians initiate treatment with a new technology, the local Primary Care Trust (PCT) must fund it. The evaluation of drugs typically focuses on the cost-effectiveness of the intervention for sub-groups of patients, and guidance is based on the cost per quality-adjusted life year (QALY). Although NICE denies the existence of a 'cut' value, appraisals with results below £20 000 per QALY get approved, those between £20 000 and £30 000 per QALY are discussed and usually supported and those in excess of £30 000 per QALY may fail.

This rationing function of NICE can be contentious, especially when patient groups with and without links to drug companies use the media to advocate special treatment of their members.[12] However, NICE's function is essential because, without it, clinical discretion would lead to variation in practice and patient access to new technologies. Rather than have such anarchy, the solution now accepted by the English, Welsh and Northern Irish governments is that NICE should take the best evidence that is available and evaluate the clinical and cost-effectiveness of interventions so as to ensure that resources are targeted at patients efficiently.

As a consequence, standard-setting is national and local discretion in principle is minimal. In reality, there is uneven take-up of new technologies approved by NICE[13] and this local discretion is leading to inequality in access to care and a failure to use what NICE regards as cost-effective interventions for designated sub-groups of the population. Thus NICE, itself introduced to reduce postcode rationing created by variations in local decision-making, is creating a new form of postcode prescribing because of differences in clinical take-up of the technologies they have appraised. Such variation is common-place in clinical practice and should be better managed to reduce inequality in access to care and inefficiency in failure to take up what is cost-effective.

INCENTIVISING NATIONAL GUIDANCE

'You can lead a horse to water, but you can't make it drink' is an appropriate aphorism to describe the problem of translating evidence into practice in healthcare. Advocacy of integration in healthcare and social care, and increased investment in secure units and alcohol and drug treatment services, have been policy 'priorities' for decades. For instance, 30 years ago the Department of Health emphasised:

> Close contact between the Health Service and Social Services departments, and between both and voluntary organisations, is of course of supreme importance in providing an effective service within the resources available.[14]

Politicians and policy-makers rediscover the problem of lack of joined-up service delivery at regular intervals. Similarly, 'solutions' are proffered for this problem. These solutions involve incentivising either to the patient and/or to the provider.

Incentivising patients

There is renewed advocacy of devolving budgets to the patients, not necessarily in cash but in kind, e.g. vouchers for patients to use to buy services from competing public and private agencies that are appropriate for their care.[15] This is a derivative of work done by Davies, Challis and colleagues in the Personal Social Services Research Unit (PSSRU) at Kent University several decades ago. Their work explored issues around the use of cash by elderly patients to purchase services and it demonstrated that such policies were feasible at reasonable costs and perhaps with some improvements in patient outcomes.[16] The issue is, would ear-marked vouchers allocated to mental health patients in the community or to their carers lead to more efficiently integrated service delivery? For instance, would the carers of dementia patients be able to mobilise improved care if they had cash to buy services, rather than inefficient public and private agencies providing care in kind? The PSSRU findings, elaborated recently, demonstrate scope for efficiency gains for patients.[17]

Incentivising providers

Another way in which efficient and integrated service delivery can be incentivised is with the use of provider incentives. This can take several forms. For instance, the English Department of Health is proposing to create a uniform pricing system for all mental health institutions. This involves the likely extension to mental hospitals, over the next three years, of the payment by results (PbR) system that currently applies to acute hospitals.[18] This is a bold decision as many countries have national hospital tariff systems like PbR (usually called diagnostic-related groups (DRGs) elsewhere) but exclude the mental health sector.

One reason for the exclusion of mental health activity from DRG systems is that the national tariff is usually fixed in relation to average system-wide costs and in psychiatry the variation around the mean can be considerable. However, such pricing systems make financial characteristics of Trusts more transparent and may induce them to be more efficient in their use of resources. There are also plans to extend PbR to the 'third sector', so that when, for instance, PCTs are commissioning services from private for profit and charitable providers, trading will be bound by a national tariff for services purchased.

In addition to incentivising hospitals, the Government is increasingly seeking to improve the service delivery of physicians and their teams. For instance, the expensive and liberally funded 2004 general practitioners (GPs) contract raised practitioners' salaries to an average above £100 000 by incentivising through a quality outcomes framework (QOF) for the provision of a range of services, including one mental health item.[19] The performance of GP practices in relation to these targets earned them points, each worth £125. The success of the QOF surprised Government. It seems, although evaluation is poor, that practices changed performance rapidly to earn QOF points, and consequently Government estimates of the cost were exceeded by £250 million.[20] Target payment systems such as this offer potential to incentivise change where there is a good evidence base of cost-effectiveness and where policing is thorough.

Aneurin Bevan is alleged to have argued that the only way to change the behaviour of doctors was to write a message on a cheque. The behaviour of doctors, other providers and institutions – like that of everyone else – can be influenced effectively by financial incentives. However, due caution has to be exercised if the effects of poorly designed incentives are not to produce perverse and inefficient behaviours and expenditure inflation. Like explosives, incentives have to be handled with care.

CONCLUSIONS

The rhetoric of devolving financial and provider powers to local settings has been part of the political landscape for decades. It is belied by policy-making which is increasing centralisation through detailed regulation of service standards and delivery. Whether we choose greater local autonomy or increasing centralisation and accountability, it is essential to recognise the limited evidence base that informs both policy-making and the medical practice. There are many unknowns, but this does not prevent frantic waves of 'redisorganisations' of policy and practice. These should be evaluated: reform is a social experiment which may damage patients and their carers, however good the intentions of well-meaning policy-makers.

The drive for value for money in the public sector and accountability for the £80 billion spent on the NHS is creating national standards and incentive systems. A decision to move away from these in a *National* Health Service is unlikely. If it were to occur, one might hope that the knowledge base would be systematically reviewed and subsequently carefully augmented in relation to what works for patients. 'What works' would be expressed in terms of clinical and cost effectiveness and how incentives could be used to induce efficient behaviour. The cost of creating knowledge can be high, but the cost of ignorance for patients and taxpayers may be even higher.

REFERENCES

1 Williams A. Need as a demand concept (with special reference to health). In: Culyer AJ, editor. *Economic Policies and Social Goals: aspects of public choice.* London: Martin Robertson; 1974.

2 Maynard A. Evidence based medicine: an incomplete method for informing treatment choices. *Lancet.* 1997; **349**: 126–8.

3 Maynard A, editor. *The Public–Private Mix for Health.* Oxford: Radcliffe Publishing; 2005.

4 Skrabanek P, McCormick JS. *Follies and Fallacies in Medicine.* Glasgow: Taragon Press; 1989.

5 British Medical Association. *Clinical Evidence Concise.* London: BMJ Publishing; 2005.

6 Geddes J, Freemantle N, Harrison P, *et al.* Atypical antipsychotics in the treatment of schizophrenia: systematic overview and meta-regression analysis. *BMJ.* 2000; **321**: 1371–6.

7 Waxman WE. The lessons of Vioxx: drug safety and sales. *New Engl J Med.* 2005; **352**: 2576–8.

8 Chalmers I. Biomedical research: are we getting value for money? *Significance.* 2006; **December**: 172–5.

9 Chalmers I. Trying to do more good than harm in policy and practice: the role of rigorous, transparent, up-to-date evaluations. *Ann Am Acad Pol Soc Sci.* 2003; **589**: 22–40.

10 Moynihan R, Cassels A. *Selling Sickness.* New South Wales: Allen and Unwin; 2005.

11 Angell M. *The Truth about the Drug Companies: how they deceive us and what to do about it.* New York: Random House; 2004.

12 Maynard A. Transparency in health technology appraisals. *BMJ.* 2007; **334**: 594–5.

13 Sheldon TA, Cullum N, Dawson D, *et al.* What's the evidence that NICE guidance has been implemented? *BMJ.* 2004; **329**: 999.

14 Department of Health and Social Security. *Priorities in Health and Personal Social Services.* London: HMSO; 1976, p. 58.

15 Le Grand J. *From Target to Market.* In press.

16 Challis DJ, Davies BP. *Matching Resources to Needs in Long Term Care.* London: Gower; 1986.

17 Knapp M, Challis D, Fernandez JL, *et al.*, editors. *Long Term Care: Matching Resources to Needs.* London: Ashgate; 2005.

18 Department of Health. *Options for the Future of Payment by Results 2007–10: a consultation document.* London: Department of Health; 2007.

19 Maynard A, Bloor K. Do those who pay the piper call the tune? *Health Policy Matters.* 2003; **8**. Available at: www.york.ac.uk/healthsciences/pubs/hpmindex.htm.

20 House of Commons. *Workforce Planning: Select Committee on Health.* London: House of Commons; 2007. HC 171.

CHAPTER 4

New ways of working in mental health services

CHRISTINE VIZE

New ways of working (NWW) is about developing new, enhanced and changed roles for mental health staff, and redesigning systems and processes to support staff to deliver effective, person-centred care in a way that is personally, financially and organisationally sustainable. This chapter will explore the evolution and state of development of NWW, the changes it can make to services and the service user experience, and its future potential.

WHAT ARE NEW WAYS OF WORKING?

The core of a mental health service is its staff, and those staff can be developed in three ways: existing staff can work differently, existing staff can be trained in additional skills, and different roles can be developed to bring new people into the workforce. Examples of these new ways of working (NWW) are given below. These staff can then form a capable team if they are deployed within a service model attuned to the needs of its users, supported by good systems (particularly information systems) and adequate resources, and embedded within a values-driven organisational culture with leadership and effective team working modelled at all levels.

This may sound like a pipe dream to many service users, carers and staff, but it is the vision for NWW, and for reasons which will be explored in this chapter, it is the only way forward for a 21st-century mental health service which wants to be fit for purpose. NWW is producing some encouraging results, but it also faces significant challenges. Its strength is that it is being driven by practitioners themselves who can see its potential for enhancing the quality of care, and for empowering service users and carers.

WHY WERE NEW WAYS OF WORKING NEEDED?

The term 'new ways of working' has been used in the Health Service for a while. In mental health, the main developments have been since 2003. Two national conferences about the role of the psychiatrist at the beginning of that year[1] focused attention on difficulties in the profession, including:

➤ significant problems with recruitment and retention, leading to high spending on locum staff and poorer services to users
➤ high and increasing levels of work-related stress and burnout amongst psychiatrists, as demonstrated by research[2]
➤ attracting new entrants to the specialty, related to what they observed of the consultant role during medical training
➤ an average consultant caseload of nearly 300
➤ an increase in the demands placed on psychiatrists, particularly for clinical governance, risk management and training
➤ a reduction in the service availability of doctors in training as a result of the New Deal and the Working Time Directive, with knock-on effects for consultants.

Following the conference, Antony Sheehan, Chief Executive of the National Institute for Mental Health in England [NIMHE]/Mental Health Policy Lead and Mike Shooter, the then President of the Royal College of Psychiatrists, set up a National Steering Group and two working groups to develop new ways of working to tackle these issues. It was clear that services needed to move away from a model where the consultant was deemed to have ultimate responsibility for everything, and where he or she was often referred to as the 'Responsible Medical Officer' when the Mental Health Act was not involved, so underlining this role. Consultants needed smaller personal caseloads in order to spend more time supporting and advising others, giving input in the most complex cases, and participating and leading governance and development.

Since 2003, more proactive mental health providers have realised that there are other drivers for NWW. The Government intends to extend Payment by Results (PbR) to mental health by 2008, and traditional methods of working, with decision-making and responsibility concentrated in the most senior staff to whom others need to refer, are going to prove too expensive and inflexible to enable Trusts to operate within the tariff. All organisations will have to invest in Connecting for Health, but the potential benefits in terms of service efficiency and enhanced quality of care will not be realised if organisations simply substitute computer for paper but keep their systems and processes the same. Service users and carers want choice in how they access care, as well as where it is provided and by whom. The Increasing Access to Psychological Therapies programme and the opportunities afforded by Foundation Trust status offer a variety of possibilities for extending and enhancing service provision, but it will only be those providers with a flexible, responsive workforce who will be in a position to take advantage of them. NWW across the primary–secondary care interface is essential if providers are to survive when Practice Based Commissioning really gets underway. The amended Mental Health Act[3] provides opportunities for developing enhanced roles for staff, and the White Paper *Our Health, Our Care, Our Say*[4] and the promised reforms to the Care Programme Approach[5] offer further impetus for change.

HOW HAS THE NEW WAYS OF WORKING INITIATIVE DEVELOPED?

Nationally, the NWW programme has been co-ordinated by the NIMHE National Workforce Programme, now part of the Care Services Improvement Partnership (CSIP). The National Steering Group continues to meet, and there are now multi-professional sub-groups, with strong service user and carer involvement, looking at what NWW means for each profession (occupational therapists and other allied health professionals, nurses, psychiatrists, psychologists, social workers and primary care). From these sub-groups, common themes are emerging as the focus for further work, including teamworking and leadership, non-medical prescribing, accountability and responsibility and continuity of care.

Some pump-priming money was provided for a variety of pilot projects in Trusts throughout the country, including the development of specialist inpatient and community consultant roles, redesign of care pathways and processes, enhanced roles for nurses including prescribing and nurse-led services, learning sets on leadership, multi-disciplinary assessment clinics, redefining the role of the consultant psychiatrist and new models of working with primary care. The pilot projects initially focused on services for adults of working age, but the principles of NWW apply to all types of teams, operating across the lifespan and across primary and secondary care, and the national work has expanded to reflect this. There are currently 10 sites testing out NWW in child and adolescent mental health services. Many pilots are now being incorporated into mainstream service development, and similar work is taking place in many other Trusts, summarised in the 'achievements' section.

Two significant reports have been produced[6,7] with detailed action plans which are being implemented, and the first *Joint Guidance on the Employment of Consultant Psychiatrists*.[8] A third report, with more supporting material, is due in 2007. Dozens of workshops and seminars have been held, organised by the national team, service user leads, Regional Development Centres, professional colleges, Trusts and others.

EXAMPLES OF NEW WAYS OF WORKING

Consultant psychiatrists in any type of community service who have embraced NWW will be working with a model of distributed responsibility within their teams, with each team member clearly taking responsibility for the care, treatment and advice that she or he provides. The model of leadership within the team is likely to be dispersed, with no automatic assumption that the consultant is the sole leader. When the consultant is away for any reason, the team will continue to function effectively with no or minimal reliance on a covering consultant. The consultant role is likely to involve:

➤ being readily available for advice or support to team members and colleagues in primary care, including advice by phone or email

➤ not seeing service users routinely in outpatient clinics, but seeing them when needed, at the request of the service user, carer, general practitioner or care co-ordinator, and often with the latter

➤ freed-up time to see those with the most complex needs, and being able to respond in a timely fashion when called upon

➤ increased emphasis on the training of others, including for example non-medical prescribers

➤ contributing to service development and clinical governance

➤ effective use of available technology – email, electronic diary, BlackBerry or PDA.

The consultant may provide telephone consultations where appropriate, or be able to email service users. She or he may participate in joint assessments of new referrals with other members of the team.

Inpatient NWW has included the development of alternatives to the traditional ward round, almost universally hated by inpatients, and the more effective use of care planning across the care pathway. In some areas, consultants have specialised in either inpatient or community work. This is sometimes called the 'functional localisation model'. Wards with dedicated inpatient consultants have shown improved teamworking and leadership, provide more therapeutic time with patients, and have better outcomes for service users in terms of satisfaction and lengths of stay. The morale of staff, particularly inpatient nurses, has improved alongside their job satisfaction.

An example of enhancing and developing the skills of existing staff is the development of non-medical prescribing. This involves training which has thus far been mostly undertaken by nurses, during which they are supervised by a consultant psychiatrist – a new way of working in itself, as psychiatrists have traditionally only trained other psychiatrists. These nurse prescribers have until recently been able to agree a Clinical Management Plan with the service user and an independent prescriber (usually the consultant psychiatrist), which has enabled them to prescribe for the service user within the parameters of the plan, which may include changing doses or drugs. From 2006 the regulations have also permitted independent prescribing. This has yet to be used widely in mental health, but there are good models in other specialities to learn from. Pharmacists in mental health, although still scarce in the workforce, are keen to collaborate in non-medical prescribing and to contribute to medicines management in multi-disciplinary teams.

The new roles that have been developed include those for which there have been national programmes – such as gateway workers, graduate mental health workers, support time and recovery workers and community development workers – and those auspiced by provider organisations themselves. The latter have worked with their local universities to set up training for a variety of assistant, associate and advanced practitioner roles, all of which can be used to free up other staff. Assistant and associate practitioners or mental health workers can take on support work with service users and contribute to care co-ordination or act as associate care co-ordinators, providing more contact time for those who need it. Advanced practitioners can take on some of the tasks previously done exclusively by medics, such as physical assessment and the management of psychiatric emergencies in the inpatient unit. The advantages of this are that these practitioners are generally onsite, rather than on-call, and the development of these enhanced skills by nursing staff can help Trusts to avoid paying punitive on-call rates to junior doctors, and to deploy their resources more effectively.

WHAT HAVE NEW WAYS OF WORKING ACHIEVED SO FAR?

A survey of English secondary mental health providers (Mental Health Trusts and Primary Care Trusts) was carried out in the summer of 2006. Two-thirds (49) have replied and been analysed by the time of writing. The results show:

➤ 63% have discussed the *Final Report on New Ways of Working* at Trust Board and Executive Team level, and 37% have an explicit action plan to implement its recommendations, which cover the development of NWW for all professions

➤ 55% have endorsed a vision of the roles and responsibilities of consultant psychiatrists at Board level. Stating explicitly that the consultant psychiatrist does not have overall responsibility for the team's activities, or the team caseload, is an important prerequisite for developing teams and distributing responsibility amongst team members

➤ 78% said that the average multi-disciplinary team in the Trust would have an idea about what NWW is about

➤ 59% have current NWW projects, and 55% have projects in the planning stage. In 30% of cases, these projects are in partnership with other organisations, such as primary care or the non-statutory sector

➤ 82% were aware of the Joint Guidance on the Employment of Consultant Psychiatrists,[9] and 80% look at the potential for developing NWW when doing their annual job plan reviews

➤ 37% had some consultants specialising in acute inpatient care, or in the acute care pathway (inpatient and crisis work)

➤ 49% had done some analysis of what consultant psychiatrists do in their outpatient clinics. These surveys have led psychiatrists themselves to reorganise outpatient care, by demonstrating that the traditional model of routine outpatient appointments, often over many years, is inefficient and insufficiently responsive

➤ 78% said that they would not automatically fill a consultant vacancy with a locum. This indicates a shift in thinking from a few years ago, when a locum, often from an agency at vast expense, was the automatic response to a vacancy, creating significant financial difficulties and often resulting in poorer outcomes for service users than more creative use of other members of the team or other teams.

A range of guidance, tools and information has been produced[10] and much more supporting material will be made available in 2007. The General Medical Council has amended its guidance to recognise that psychiatrists work in teams with distributed responsibility, rather than responsibility simply being delegated from them. The amendments to the Mental Health Act 1983 will be in accordance with NWW principles. For the first time, the Royal College of Psychiatrists and NHS employers have agreed joint guidance on the employment of consultant psychiatrists. NWW is being considered in the pilot work for Payment by Results, and in the national review of the Care Programme Approach. National Workforce Projects have commissioned two pilot projects to examine NWW in relation to compliance with the Working

Time Directive for junior doctors in 2009. The Healthcare Commission will include questions on NWW in its Staff Survey from 2008.

HOW DO NEW WAYS OF WORKING IMPACT ON SERVICE USERS, CARERS AND STAFF?

Service users and carers may find that the elements of their care plans can be delivered through contact with fewer members of staff, where those staff have additional training, for example in psychological interventions or prescribing. They may find that they need to see a psychiatrist less often, but should find one more easily accessible when needed, and be able to see them as frequently as necessary when they are acutely unwell. They will have choices in the way they and the staff communicate. A greater number of staff used to dealing with medication, including an increasing number of clinical pharmacists, will mean that service users and carers can be better informed about medication and the choices thereof. Improved working across the interface between primary and secondary care will mean that side effects and other physical health difficulties can be more systematically monitored, and will increase the opportunities for that interface to become a continuum, which service users can move along in either direction according to their needs. They should benefit from improved communication and teamworking, including timely decision-making.

When service users are admitted to hospital, they may find that the consultant working with the inpatient team is different from the one working with the community team. This can feel difficult for inpatients, and the best arrangements like this have worked to improve continuity of care across the inpatient and community services, with workers who bridge the two, and continued involvement of the community team to help plan for discharge from the time of admission.

Other people may never become users of a secondary mental health service as they would have done in the past. Their needs may be met entirely in the primary care setting, perhaps through the intervention of a primary care mental health team offering group or individual psychological therapies or psycho-education, possibly with the aid of additional advice from the secondary care team.

NWW impacts on both the shape of a mental health team, and the way in which the team members work. Instead of a team requiring a certain number of professionals from each of the traditional groups, NWW – through a tool that has been developed called the Creating Capable Teams Approach – looks at the needs of the population served by the team, and then the competencies required to meet them. The actual composition of teams will therefore differ according to who has which skills and competencies, and they will not be formed around consultant psychiatrist posts as often happened in the past. Within the team, more supportive work may be carried out by trained but not professionally qualified staff, freeing up the qualified staff for more specialised interventions such as psychological therapies. Responsibility will be distributed amongst the team members, rather than the ultimate responsibility for the care of all the service users on the team's caseload residing with the consultant psychiatrist, as often happened in the past. This will result in a more robust approach to risk assessment and management. However, the psychiatrist will be readily accessible, and team members may be able to book service users in directly to see the consultant. The team may do joint assessments, with other team members or colleagues from other services including primary care, and specialist drug and alcohol services.

WHAT ARE THE CHALLENGES IN DEVELOPING NEW WAYS OF WORKING?

NWW is what it says – ways of working – rather than a single service model or structure which has to be adopted. It recognises that services catering for different types of needs, across the lifespan, with different demographics and geography, will need different configurations to manage their task most effectively, but that the underlying principles relating to using the skills of the workforce in the most productive way are common. It is about achieving cultural change – a shift in the way teams think about themselves, the skills of the individuals within them, and the reasons they are there – and cultural change is a difficult thing to achieve, and to measure to know you have achieved it.

There are challenges at all levels in developing NWW. Nationally the means of disseminating information, and particularly sharing good practice, are not well developed, and it remains to be seen whether Foundation Trusts will be less willing in future to share information and experience with prospective competitors. Education and training budgets are under increasing pressure across the country as the NHS tries to deliver its promise of achieving financial balance, and it is often training for new or enhanced roles that is most vulnerable.

At Trust level, the recognition of, the need for and the development of NWW is variable. Unfortunately the drive for Foundation Trust status and the pressure to achieve and maintain financial stability are distracting from the NWW agenda in many places, with inadequate realisation that all these aims can work together – it should be 'both, and' rather than 'either/or'. Workforce redesign, rather than expansion, is the clear message from the Department of Health regarding what is in store for the next five years, but this is not always being translated into developing NWW.

At individual and professional level there are concerns that NWW is a way of cutting costs or 'dumbing down' the skill-mix of the workforce. Some psychiatrists are concerned at the prospect of other professions taking on parts of what was previously their role, and other non-medical professionals sometimes complain that this is a way to get doctors on the cheap, and that if they are doing the work of doctors they should have parity of pay with them. In some teams and organisations there is 'change fatigue' due to constant re-organisations over the past few years, and at these times staff retreat into what they know, even if they also realise it is not the best way to run a service. Some staff may feel that there is nothing 'new' about NWW, and that it just reflects the way they have worked for many years, so where that is the case the challenge is to turn cynicism into a desire to disseminate good practice.

There are some problems around continuity of care where NWW has resulted in quite a high level of specialisation of teams. Further work is needed to ensure service users have a more seamless experience, but generally it is significant that the challenges are perhaps least in persuading service users and carers of the merits of NWW. A few may have reservations about losing routine appointments with 'their' psychiatrist, in the same way as they have done to a large extent with 'their' GP, but improvements in accessibility and timeliness of response from staff with a wider range of skills make those who have experienced good NWW influential advocates for the cause.

WHAT OPPORTUNITIES DO NEW WAYS OF WORKING OFFER FOR THE FUTURE?

The providers of mental health services in the future will need to have a workforce that is skilled, flexible and adaptable to provide the services that service users and carers, through commissioners, need and want. Those services will have to demonstrate that they are both effective, in terms of outcomes for service users and carers, and efficient in their use of resources. Many services at present are still bound by traditional ideas of which profession has to do what, and improvements in service delivery are often very slow to achieve, in contrast to the fast pace of organisational and structural change. In a lot of cases, service development is hindered by the lack of quality local information. It is difficult to see how the transformation that will be required can take place without NWW, and perfectly possible to see how those teams, services and organisations that are slow or resistant to NWW will at some point be overtaken by events – losing work to competitors or becoming financially unsustainable.

NWW is developing well in many places, but nowhere can it be said to be embedded across an entire organisation, except perhaps the smallest Primary Care Trust (PCT) providers of mental health services. Perhaps when it is, the measure of success will be that the term will not be necessary any more – NWW will simply be the most sensible, logical way to deliver services. To get to that point, where it is part of mainstream thinking, requires several things:

➤ more time, as achieving cultural change is a gradual process, and because people rightly want to be convinced by evidence, which takes time to emerge and is complex to evaluate

➤ continued support at a national level, to facilitate shared learning and the development of national guidance, and occasionally solutions, where providers are coming across common difficulties

➤ leadership and vision, from national to organisational to team level, to spot and develop the myriad opportunities for making real improvements, and to see the links between the different national agendas that can be made at local level, too

➤ courage from those leaders, to not allow themselves to be deflected from the goal by short-termism and fire-fighting, the need for which would be largely eliminated by achieving the goal

➤ development of the requisite skills and capacity within organisations to foster leadership and team development

➤ more effective commissioning of mental health services, including an understanding of governance and development needs

➤ inclusion of measures of NWW in performance indicators, to give NWW explicit endorsement, more exposure and parity with other measures of quality and outcomes

➤ the routine use of 'intelligent information' from team level upwards, to inform the development and evaluation of NWW throughout organisations, and to disseminate learning.

And finally, NWW needs to be linked much more explicitly to two other powerful drivers of change in the workforce and working practice – Connecting for Health and Foundation Trust status. Perhaps it will be that, by becoming members and Governors of Foundation Trusts, service users and carers demanding NWW could be most powerfully articulated.

REFERENCES

1 National Working Group on New Roles for Psychiatrists. *New Roles for Psychiatrists.* London: Department of Health; 2004. Gateway ref: 2710. Available at: www.dh.gov.uk/ PublicationsAndStatistics/Publications/PublicationsPolicyAndGuidance/ PublicationsPolicyAndGuidanceArticle/fs/en?CONTENT_ID=4073490&chk =4K2Tni.

2 Mears A, Pajak S, Kendall T, *et al. Consultant Psychiatrists' Working Patterns: is a progressive approach the key to staff retention?* 2004. Available at: http://pb.rcpsych.org/ cgi/content/abstract/28/7/251.

3 Amended Mental Health Bill. 2006. Available at: www.dh.gov.uk/PolicyAndGuidance/ HealthAndSocialCareTopics/MentalHealth/MentalHealthList/fs/en?CONTENT_ ID=4001816&chk=Tg1/Et.

4 Department of Health. *Our Health, Our Care, Our Say.* London: Department of Health. 2006; Gateway ref: 7191. Available at: www.dh.gov.uk/PublicationsAndStatistics/Publications/ PublicationsPolicyAndGuidance/PublicationsPolicyAndGuidanceArticle/fs/en? CONTENT_ID=4139925&chk=Vixg2n.

5 Care Services Improvement Partnership. *Reviewing the Care Programme Approach.* London: Department of Health; 2006. Available at: www.dh.gov.uk/Consultations/ LiveConsultations/LiveConsultationsArticle/fs/en?CONTENT_ID=4140544&chk =bPo0X6.

6 National Steering Group for New Ways of Working. *Guidance on New Ways of Working for Psychiatrists in a Multi-disciplinary and Multi-agency Context.* London: Department of Health; 2004. Gateway ref: 3304. Available at: www.dh.gov.uk/ PublicationsAndStatistics/Publications/PublicationsPolicyAndGuidance/ PublicationsPolicyAndGuidanceArticle/fs/en?CONTENT_ID=4087352&chk =01RXVr.

7 Royal College of Psychiatrists, National Institute for Mental Health in England. *New Ways of Working for Psychiatrists: enhancing effective, person-centred services through new ways of working in multi-disciplinary and multi-agency contexts.* Final report 'but not the end of the story'. London: Department of Health; 2005. Gateway ref: 5067. Available at: www.dh.gov.uk/PublicationsAndStatistics/Publications/ PublicationsPolicyAndGuidance/PublicationsPolicyAndGuidanceArticle/fs/ en?CONTENT_ID=4122342&chk=RbKb2y.

8 Royal College of Psychiatrists, NHS Confederation, National Mental Health Partnership. *Joint Guidance on the Employment of Consultant Psychiatrists.* London: Department of Health; 2005. Gateway ref: 5068. Available at: www.dh.gov. uk/PublicationsAndStatistics/Publications/PublicationsPolicyAndGuidance/ PublicationsPolicyAndGuidanceArticle/fs/en?CONTENT_ID=4122352 &chk=CWEIUX.

9 Ibid.

10 Royal College of Psychiatrists. Gateway ref: 5067. Op. cit.

CHAPTER 5

More than black and white: mental health services provided to people from black and minority ethnic communities

SARAH ELLIX and KALA SUBBUSWAMY

Research over 30 years has established that there are disturbing links between poor treatment/outcomes, and differentials in ethnic origin within many of Britain's public institutions, leading in 1999 to the MacPherson report's unveiling of the concept of 'institutional racism'.[1] The mental health system is no exception, but the adverse treatment of black people within it, as within the criminal justice system,[2] is of particular concern because those who access it are not only likely to be relatively powerless and liable to isolation, but they are also more likely to be misunderstood and/or feared by wider society, and more susceptible to abuse.

In this chapter, we will be using the terms 'black' and 'black and minority ethnic (BME)', referring primarily to people with African, Caribbean, Asian, or dual/multiple heritages. This also includes people who regard themselves as Black British or British Asian. There are issues of inequality and discrimination for some White ethnic groups, and we certainly do not exclude them from our analysis. However, figures available suggest that the greatest inequalities and disadvantages within the mental health system are still experienced by non-White ethnic groups. The terms 'mental health survivor' and 'service user' will also be used. 'Service user' is the currently favoured term in most government literature, but we also use 'survivor', to indicate people's survival through the discrimination, exclusion and prejudice that they often experience in society because of their label of mental illness, as well as their survival through everyday emotional and mental struggles.

In 2005, the Government published its *Delivering Race Equality in Mental Health Care (DRE)*[3] strategy. The vision of *DRE*, which is expected to deliver on outcomes by 2010, is:

- less fear of mental health services among BME communities
- increased satisfaction with services
- a reduction in the rate of admission of people from BME communities to psychiatric inpatient units
- a reduction in the disproportionate rates of compulsory detention of BME service users in inpatient units
- fewer violent incidents that are secondary to inadequate treatment of mental illness
- a reduction in the use of seclusion in BME groups
- the prevention of deaths in mental health services following physical intervention
- more BME service users reaching self-reported states of recovery
- a reduction in the ethnic disparities found in prison populations
- a more balanced range of effective therapies, such as peer support services and psychotherapeutic and counselling treatments, as well as pharmacological interventions that are culturally appropriate and effective
- a more active role for BME communities and black service users in the training of professionals, in the development of mental health policy, and in the planning and provision of services
- a workforce and organisation capable of delivering appropriate and responsive mental health services to BME communities.

The publication of *DRE* was partly prompted by the inquiry into the death of David Bennett in the Norvic Clinic (a medium-security unit), in 1998. This followed an earlier report, published in 1995 on the deaths of three African-Caribbean patients at Broadmoor Hospital,[4] the recommendations of which chime strongly with those from the Bennett inquiry.

David Bennett was African-Caribbean, and had been diagnosed with schizophrenia in 1985. He was subject to racist abuse from another patient on 30 October 1998, following an argument where each man struck the other, and David was removed from the ward. The staff failed to discuss the issue of racism with the other patient, and David's subsequent and unfair removal from the ward appears to have agitated him, leading to his hitting a nurse. David was subsequently held in a prone position (face down) for approximately 25 minutes. During the struggle he collapsed and was later pronounced dead at hospital.

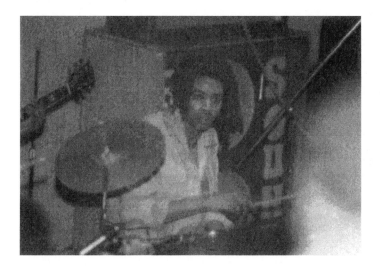

FIGURE 5.1 David 'Rocky' Bennett. Reproduced with permission.

It is significant, yet disturbing, to note that in 1993 David Bennett wrote an eloquent letter to the Head of Nursing at the Norvic Clinic, which indicated a personal and expert awareness of issues affecting his care.

> As you know, there are half a dozen black boys in this clinic. I don't know if you have realised that there are no Africans on your staff at the moment. We feel there should be at least two black persons in the medical or social work staff. For the obvious reasons of security and contentment for all concerned, please do your best to remedy this situation.[5]
>
> **Reproduced with permission.**

David received a reply stating there had been no black applicants for years, and by the time of the inquiry it appeared little further positive action had been taken to address his legitimate concerns. It is evident that the service, the community and society have lost a great advocate here, as well as a sensitive human being; for his family, the sense of loss must be insurmountable.

In a small, national consultation by the authors on the state of current mental health services to black and minority groups, Michael Howlett of The Zito Trust offered the following powerful statement:

> The social and healthcare implications of the DRE, and the lessons to be learned from the inquiry into the death of David Bennett, highlight the importance of not only arriving at an understanding of what is going on within our mental health

(and prison) services, but also what realistically can be done to act on that understanding to bridge the divide which currently exists in the many different experiences people have of the care offered to (or withdrawn from) them.

Initiatives which are explicit and practical in terms of design and delivery have the power to bring people together for a common purpose. These initiatives must, however, tackle the unconscious agenda, which lies at the heart of racism and many other forms of discrimination. Some of the motivation here will be based on fear arising from stereotypes. The core of the problem is deep-rooted and complex. Likewise, the process, which leads to change, must also be sufficiently probing as well as properly resourced.

Organisations including The Zito Trust, the Sainsbury Centre for Mental Health, the Joseph Rowntree Foundation, and Mind, have long asserted the need for far-reaching, radical changes to improve the experiences of black people who need to use mental health services. Despite this, the recent *Count Me In* national census of people in psychiatric inpatient wards found that people from BME communities (particularly people of African/African-Caribbean heritage) are still over-represented in psychiatric admissions, including detentions under the Mental Health Act 1983, and still report more negative experiences in the mental health system itself.[6,7]

Mental health survivors from black communities, and their carers, frequently report negative experiences of mainstream mental health services, including that services stereotype them, offer control rather than assistance, and assume their intellectual inferiority, especially if English is not their first language.[8] Other themes include: experiences of isolation and alienation, not feeling understood or respected, and lack of acknowledgement of racism – both past and present.[9,10]

Two important questions arise here for those with responsibility to provide, deliver, plan and develop such services: Why have the inequalities for black people experiencing mental ill-health not yet been reduced? and How can mental health services and the wider community create real and lasting change in the future?

In their challenging and thought-provoking chapter in this book, 'Race and mental health: there is more to race than racism', originally published in the *British Medical Journal* in 2006, Swaran P Singh and Tom Burns criticise the contention that mental health services are institutionally discriminatory and racist.[11] They suggest a number of other explanations, including (disputed) evidence of differential patterns of psychiatric illness in different ethnic groups; variations in social/economic circumstances, and differences in help-seeking behaviours leading to different routes into service provision.

Singh and Burns also point to a 'spiral of downward engagement' between black service users, their carers and mental health services, leading inevitably to more coercive responses from services. They seem to gloss over the complex reasons for this, implying that 'alienation and distrust of statutory services among inner city black youth' and the concept of institutional racism itself are to blame. However, their criticisms of the label of institutional racism seem to stem from a misunderstanding of what the term truly means.

It is our understanding that wherever there are processes or patterns, systems or structures, that have disproportionate effects on certain sections of the population, this is institutional discrimination. Where this impact is negative in disproportionate degrees against certain BME communities, this is unlawful discrimination under *Race Relations* legislation. If there are practices within psychiatry that are producing adverse outcomes for certain groups, systems should be properly checked for such influences. There is no room to hide through complacency, or by passing the buck to the community itself or to the service user. The fact that there will always be a power imbalance between service users and professionals requires professionals to take more proactive responsibility for removing these barriers, in order to provide more appropriate care

WHAT IS IT ABOUT THE MENTAL HEALTH SYSTEM THAT CREATES (OR FAILS TO PREVENT) RACIST OUTCOMES?

A western model of mental health and mental health problems

As Fernando[12] says, 'statutory mental health services [in Britain] have continued to use a model that encapsulates most mental health problems as essentially medical illnesses based on traditional western European psychiatry', giving a number of examples about the nature of 'self' and the relationship between the individual and the collective, which are at odds with other cultural world views.[13,14] The dominance of the medical model has profound practical consequences on communication, understanding and feelings of respect between mental health professionals, black service users, their families/carers and wider communities.

Avoidance and denial of issues of racism, discrimination, power and abuse

The impact of personal and cultural histories of racism, discrimination and oppression is a strong theme in many stories of black people within the mental health system.[15] Within this context, similar experiences of the system itself, including the powerlessness of being subject to coercive interventions such as compulsory detention, seclusion or restraint, may compound to become unbearable. It is essential that issues of racism, discrimination, abuse/oppression and power are acknowledged and discussed within mental health services. However, many staff within the system feel strong anxieties about talking openly about race and culture, let alone exploring racism.[16] This could be one of the reasons why 'cultural competence' or 'cultural awareness' training has failed to really impact on the inequalities experienced by BME communities within the mental health system so far.

'Us' and 'them' culture

The prevailing attitude within modern British society, and to some degree within the mental health system, towards people with a label of mental illness is that 'they' – the mentally ill – are fundamentally different from 'us', the normal – with consequences including stigma, prejudice, discrimination/abuse, and barriers to building positive relationships. People from BME communities who experience mental health difficulties often face multiple layers of discrimination and exclusion, being seen as doubly different because they are mentally ill, and even more so, because they are black. If this is also the case within services, barriers will be even greater, and there will be less likelihood that services will provide adequate support to black service users.

> 'Brotherly love was always at a premium, and the more obvious the differences between the brothers, the less the loving.'
>
> **Braithwaite ER. *Paid Servant*. London: Bodley Head; 1962, p. 100.**

LEGISLATION PROTECTS AGAINST DISCRIMINATION, SO WHY DO INEQUALITIES STILL EXIST?

Racism is an incredibly powerful and insidious form of discrimination, either direct or indirect, open or 'stealth'. As Trevor Phillips stated recently, 'the kind of racism that smiles to your face just as it's dumping your job application in the bin marked Not White Enough'.[17] Disturbingly, there seems to be an increasing unspoken prejudice, seen most recently in *The Guardian*'s undercover report into British National Party (BNP) membership among the middle/upper classes.[18] Clearly racism should not be underestimated as a force working within healthcare.

Legislation cannot regulate against all thoughts, or indeed all actions. It can merely prohibit and try to prevent the worst kinds of discrimination. The will to change demands conscious thought and empathy, a will to reflect on one's own culture and beliefs, before trying to understand someone else's; and a radical and fundamental commitment to care.

It is clear to the authors that there is no personal escape from individual liability for the existence of institutional or structural forms of racism/discrimination. Processes and structures are products of human design and, as such, each of us holds some accountability for these unfair systems, as well as for changing them. As Ferns[19] suggests, mental health practitioners need to be 'willing to stick their necks out', to challenge and change the systems in which they work. And it should be acknowledged that everyone is institutionalised by unfair systems, those who benefit and those who do not.

This is not to disrespect, undermine or fail to acknowledge the great deal of professionalism and care provided to patients every day by committed and compassionate individuals. It is understandably hard to accept such criticism and not be defensive, particularly if you fall honourably into the category of workers described above.

This level of change can feel unsettling. Often change occurs at such a pace that there is little time to reflect properly on elements of practice, and refine our tools for future use. There must be more time and emphasis given to professional development, reflective practice, transcultural thinking and effective communication skills. This will inevitably be hard, in a system that is often forced to be reactive, and bears the brunt of increasing public pressure. And it cannot be the case that while such change takes place, vulnerable people with mental health needs, from BME communities or otherwise, are left to suffer without appropriate support.

LEICESTER: THE LOCAL PICTURE

Leicester is an incredibly diverse city and the challenges and issues described above are of great relevance here. In the 2001 census 36% of Leicester's population classed themselves as non-White, and nearly 50% of Leicester's junior school population come from ethnic minority backgrounds. It is estimated that some 8000–10 000 Somali people have arrived since the 1990s.[20] This proportion will now be even higher. Almost 6% of people under 18 years old are of dual heritage, according to the 2001 census.

There is a huge diversity of languages, cultures, religions, backgrounds, circumstances and patterns of settlement. Leicester's recent history includes the arrival of Polish and Latvian refugees in the 1940s; Indian, Pakistani and African-Caribbean workers filling the labour shortage in the 1950s; the arrival of a large East-African Asian community fleeing Idi Amin in the 1960s–70s, and the more recent Kosovan and Somali arrivals. This level of diversity is reflected in the fact that over 100 languages are spoken in the city.[21] All of the major world religions are represented, with the largest faith communities being Christian (45%), Hindu (15%), Muslim (11%) and Sikh (4%).

In terms of mental health the pattern is also mixed, with some communities over-represented and others under-represented in different parts of the service. People of African and Caribbean descent are over-represented in assessments under the Mental Health Act 1983, in inpatient admissions generally, and in a range of mental health services locally, from assertive outreach teams to advocacy. People from the South Asian communities are under-represented in most of the service, the one exception being day-services, with the existence of two specifically South Asian day-services projects run by the voluntary sector. Overall, people from South Asian backgrounds are also under-represented in Mental Health Act assessments, but this pattern may be changing, with younger Asian men being represented at levels commensurate with their levels in the general population, and the same trend occurring with Asian women, raising interesting questions and concerns for the future.[22]

In spite of the large black presence and influence in the city, their voices are still not as strong as they should be within the local mental health system.

> Still we see users of mental health services from BME groups sitting isolated by patients and staff on wards, because they dress differently and have no one to communicate with them in their own first language. Still we see people from BME groups being expected to fit with the predominantly western understanding, culture and diet offered by local mental health services. Still we see African Caribbean men far more likely than their white peers to be labelled with a psychotic diagnosis, to be heavily medicated, to be seen as aggressive and a potential threat, or to merit seclusion.[23]

The mental health community in Leicester, including the City Council, has responded to these challenges in a number of ways in recent years, in line with the *DRE*'s three building blocks, requiring:

➤ more appropriate and responsive services
➤ community engagement
➤ better information.

MORE APPROPRIATE AND RESPONSIVE SERVICES

Several specific BME mental health projects are supported within the city, including the Savera Resource Centre and Adhar Project, voluntary sector day-services for people from South Asian communities, and Akwaaba Ayeh, an advocacy service for people from BME communities.

> If it were not for the Advocacy Worker I do believe that I would not be out of hospital because I had great trouble articulating, for example, asking questions. They have questions for me and I have trouble answering. They were trying to confuse me and hold me down in the system, criminalizing me trying to put me into forensics and I was not aware that they were doing this to me. If it were not for the intervention of my advocacy worker I might still be in hospital. I am grateful and thankful for Akwaaba Ayeh input. I have my freedom back.[24]

The Council has supported some development work within the black mental health voluntary sector, with the employment of Community Development Workers in line with the *DRE*, and it is hoped that this will impact on mainstream mental health services by making them more accessible and appropriate for black and ethnic minority people, while also building capacity within our diverse communities to aid recovery. The Leicester City Mental Health Strategy Team has recently completed an Equality Impact Assessment on mental health information and advocacy, resulting in some key recommendations which should have a positive impact on people's access to, and relationships with, services in future.

The Council commissions both group and individual support specifically for carers of people with mental health difficulties from South Asian communities. It has also established a Carers Strategy Ethnic Minority sub-group, with the aim of discussing with frontline staff issues raised by black carers, who are then able to monitor progress on actions agreed during these discussions. The local Caring for Carers sub-group, established in response to the 1999 National Service Framework for Mental Health, has produced a *Mental Health Carers Resource Pack*, translated into the main Asian languages spoken in Leicestershire. Leicester also has a BME Care Workers Network, and in 2006 hosted the regional Reach Out conference, for carers from black communities.

The Child and Adolescent Mental Health Service (CAMHS) has a strategy built on consultation/research with the local black communities which specifically addresses the cultural and mental health needs of these young people. The concluding report recognised the national picture:

> That the extent of social exclusion amongst black and minority ethnic communities, levels of racism and racial discrimination experienced by them in public life and, more pertinently, when they come into contact with institutional agencies are key determinants of psychiatric morbidity within these groups.[25]

Within City Council Adult Services, the department's Black Workers Group and Race Equality Sub-group have provided valuable forums to discuss these issues. Leicester has also developed panels to test the quality assurance of assessment outcomes, including a specific focus on culturally appropriate care, and has implemented the Heritage Model to guide Fair Access to Care procedures.

The Heritage Model helps practitioners to work in a person-centred way, guiding them to assess care packages in relation to an individual's whole identity and to explore the factors such as race, gender, age, religion, social

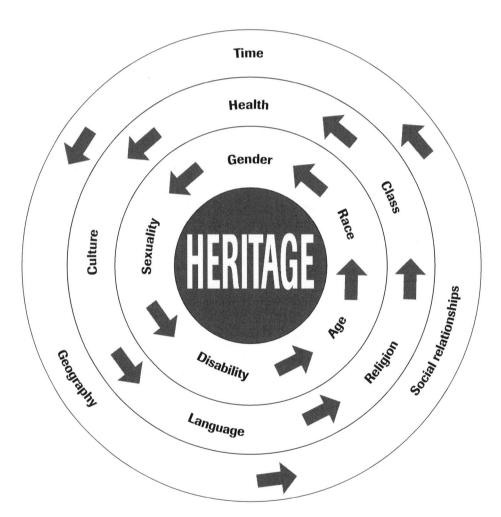

FIGURE 5.2 The Heritage Model. © 2001 Hilal Barwany for Leicester City Council (unpublished).

class, social relationships, sexual orientation and health (both physical and mental). The model acknowledges that heritage/identity is multi-faceted, fluid/dynamic, and evolves over time, meaning that assessments require regular review to ensure the continuing relevance of services.

The power of the model is that it respects and celebrates individual diversity, and explicitly embraces anti-discriminatory/anti-racist practice. It is hoped that consistent use of the model will lead to more tailored care for all service users in the future, not least those from black communities requiring access to mental healthcare.

One of the key requirements if services are to be responsive to the needs of all their communities is access to good interpretation/translation services. In Leicester these are provided for the social care and health communities mainly by Leicester City Council's Interpretation and Translation Service and the Ujala Resource Centre, part of the city's Primary Care Trust (PCT).

The Council's Interpretation and Translation Service covers over 70 languages, and through monitoring service use responds to the changing demographics in the city – for example, recently recruiting more interpreters in a number of languages such as Somali, Kurdish and Romanian, to respond to recent increases of these communities in the city.[26]

Mental health and equality training has been provided for interpreters over recent years through partnership work between the interpretation and translation providers, the City Council, the PCT, the local NHS Workforce Deanery and the local Mental Health Trust. A recent evaluation by Sure Start Highfields (Leicester) found high levels of satisfaction from staff and clients with the interpretation services they used and also showed the many positive impacts of having access to interpreters, leading to better and more sustainable relationships.

> An interpreter went into a Bengali family, she was a Bengali woman herself and there were complex problems in the family. The interpreter was able to support the family and the Sure Start professional, she had a real understanding of the culture of the family and was able to gather very sensitive information, but at the same time maintaining confidentiality within the community which was very important. Because the interpreter was bound by her professional code of conduct she was able to work within this small community confidentially.[27]

COMMUNITY ENGAGEMENT

A recent consultation project commissioned by the City Council, undertaken by Akwaaba Ayeh, reiterated the urgent need to improve our engagement with local BME people, especially those from African/African-Caribbean communities.[28] Carers from these communities reported struggling in isolation with huge challenges and barriers, including a lack of information about available support, a reluctance to identify themselves as 'carers', mistrust of services and community taboos in discussing mental health issues. One suggestion has been to build links with faith institutions, and this is being explored through the local Mental Health Promotion Steering Group.

There have been attempts to increase the black survivor and carer voice within mental health services, through direct consultation with existing black service user and carer groups and funding for specific consultation projects, as well as trying to support mainstream service user and carer forums to involve more people from BME communities. However, there are still major issues that mental health services need to confront, including the inaccessibility of meetings and the lack of adequate/consistent interpretation support.

BETTER INFORMATION

The City Council routinely collects and analyses data on ethnicity, gender, age and religion, with regard to use of social care services, and in our monitoring agreements with voluntary sector service providers. Mental Health Act assessments are also monitored in this way. This information does have an impact on service provision – for example, it has been taken up in recent reviews of counselling services and mental health day-services.

The local mental health community is trying, too, to improve data collection/monitoring around ethnicity, including making improvements to Mental Health Act monitoring forms and processes, and through commissioners' service-level agreements with the local Mental Health Trust. Ethnicity monitoring is becoming more embedded in all areas of practice, with cultures developing within the new services (such as crisis resolution), regular performance and progress reports, and the inclusion of issues relating to ethnicity as core.

WHAT ELSE NEEDS TO BE DONE?

➤ We need to link agendas around alternatives to the medical model, e.g. social models/recovery/person-centred approaches, and race equality expertise; and ensure that developments around alternative approaches include black voices in their discussions.

➤ We will need to encourage the black mental health service user and carer movements to have a stronger, more meaningful voice. While inclusion and participation may lead to vocal conflict, it is necessary for meaningful change.

➤ We should provide opportunities for black service users and carers to develop their skills and to be involved in the delivery of user-led training for professionals.

➤ We must provide 'safe space' for employees and service users/carers to explore and discuss issues affecting recovery or practice, including the impacts of racism. Less prescriptive processes, more room for narrative and recognising the importance of 'story-telling', could provide real opportunities to explore underlying issues/causes, and to enable genuine understanding and less fear of 'the other'.

➤ There should be sustained support for the black independent mental health sector to build its capacity, speak with a strong voice, and to work efficiently and co-operatively with other voluntary and community sector organisations and statutory services. There should be mechanisms to support and fund independent alternatives to hospital admission: e.g. service user-/voluntary sector-managed crisis houses.

➤ We should examine ways to ensure that experiences of admission do not damage relationships with BME service users; e.g. involve black advocacy workers early in the process; and, especially given the disproportionate numbers of black people coming into the system via a criminal justice route, ensure mental health institutions *feel* distinctly different from prisons.

➤ We must work to develop more representative mental health workforces; overcome issues leading to the marginalisation of black professionals in less powerful roles, while also addressing their constraints in challenging dominant cultures/models in services.

➤ We should ensure that people from black communities have good access to direct payment and individual budget schemes – these, by enabling people to commission their own care services, should provide more targeted, individualised support, guided/directed by the service user (and/or carer) themselves.

➤ We must actively promote carers' rights to assessment under the Carers Recognition and Services Act 1995 and Carers (Equal Opportunities) Act 2004 within the black community. It must be recognised, as one leading psychiatrist stated, that:

Carers are an integral part of the patient's support system . . . they are the ones with the day-to-day experience of the patient's condition . . . The carer's voice in decision-making about admission and discharge is ignored at everyone's peril – and yet, so often it is.[29]

➤ We should learn from innovative projects, including those in Bradford, Liverpool and Tower Hamlets,[30] which seem to show better outcomes for black service users. Characteristics include: less formality (e.g. it is acceptable sometimes to be late); calm/pleasant environments; approachable/non-threatening practitioners; people's linguistic/ other needs met without issue; use of clear language and avoidance of medical terminology; and the sharing of common experiences. In an ideal world, as 'mainstream' service provision improves, the need for 'separatist' and/or 'specialist' services may well diminish over time. However, as human need is diverse, the avenues for accessing services may need to remain so, too.

CONCLUSION

No challenge is impossible to overcome, given enough human will – not even the combined current stigma of racism and mental ill-health. Society itself has a role to play in supporting recovery, and will also reap the benefits of success. The Department of Health's guidance, *Action on Stigma*,[31] offers a useful starting place for promoting positive mental health and ending discrimination in employment. It is to be hoped that black survivors will benefit from a combined approach of this strategy and the better promotion of racial equality in the future.

The *DRE* could change the picture for black mental health service users and survivors by 2010. Yet this demands proper implementation; action, not rhetoric. The current reality is an illusion of progress. The news that Lord Kamlesh Patel, the national director of the Government's strategy, resigned just twelve months after his appointment, sent shockwaves through the black voluntary and community sectors, and left the *DRE* without a champion. Additionally, in a recent article by the 1990 Trust, a member of the independent inquiry panel into the death of David Bennett, Dr Richard Stone, has stated that 'not one of the recommendations . . . have [sic] been implemented since its publication'.[32]

Any improvements made to mental health service provision for the benefit of people from black and/or minority ethnic groups will arguably be beneficial to all people experiencing mental health difficulties. There are clear social, demographic, financial[33] and economic reasons for moving forward to develop the mental health service with a disposition of activism, rather than restraint.

It is time to act now, and implement change, so that today's (and tomorrow's) BME people who require access to mental health services can do so without suffering further oppression from the system itself, and can be appropriately supported to recovery. Let us accept that sometimes 'equal' does mean 'different', and that our similarities and our differences need to be acknowledged. Only when services appear and act in a genuinely culturally sensitive way will the downward spiral of engagement with some BME communities come to a halt, and will relationships begin to travel up towards equality.

REFERENCE

1 Macpherson W. *The Stephen Lawrence Inquiry: report of an inquiry by Sir William MacPherson of Cluny of the police investigation following the death of Stephen Lawrence.* London: HMSO; 1999.

2 Keith Mr Justice B. *The Report of the Zahid Mubarek Inquiry.* London: HMSO; 2006. Available at: www.zahidmubarekinquiry.org.uk

3 Department of Health. *Delivering Race Equality in Mental Health Care: an action plan for reform inside and outside services and the Government's response to the independent inquiry into the death of David Bennett.* London: Department of Health; 2005.

4 The Special Hospitals Service Authority. *Big, Black and Dangerous?: the report of the Committee of Inquiry into the death in Broadmoor Hospital of Orville Blackwood and the review of the deaths of two other Afro-Caribbean patients.* London: SHSA; 1993.

5 NHS Strategic Health Authority. Extract from the report written by Sir John Blofeld on the recommendations of the *Independent Inquiry into the death of David Bennett.* Norfolk, Suffolk and Cambridgeshire NHS Trust; December 2003.

6 Healthcare Commission, Mental Health Act Commission, Care Service Improvement Partnership. *Count Me In: results of a national census of inpatients in mental health hospitals and facilities in England and Wales.* London: Commission for Healthcare Audit and Inspection; 2005.

7 Chilvers C, Heginbotham C, Simpson J, *et al. Count Me In: the national mental health and ethnicity census 2005: service user survey.* Nottingham: Mental Health Act Commission; 2006.

8 Ferns P. Finding a way forward: a black perspective on social approaches to mental health. In: Tew J, editor. *Social Perspectives in Mental Health: developing social models to understand and work with mental distress.* London: Jessica Kingsley Publishers; 2005. pp. 129–50.

9 Keating F, Robertson D, McCulloch A, *et al. Breaking the Circles of Fear: a review of the relationship between mental health services and African and Caribbean communities.* London: Sainsbury Centre for Mental Health; 2002.

10 Westwood S, Couloute J, Desai S, *et al. Sadness in My Heart: racism and mental health.* Leicester: University of Leicester; 1989.

11 Singh SP, Burns T. Race and mental health: there is more to race than racism. *BMJ*. 2006; **333**: 648–65.

12 Fernando S. Multicultural mental health services: projects for minority ethnic communities in England. *Transcult Psychiatry*. 2005; **42(3)**: 420–36.

13 Rajamanickam B. *Transcultural Health Care Practice: core practice module*, Chapter 5: Mental health and minority ethnic groups. London: Royal College of Nursing; 2004. Available at: www.rcn.org.uk/resources/transcultural/mentalhealth/index.pp

14 Ram-Prasad C. The great divide. *Prospect*. 2006; 119. Available at: www.prospect-magazine.co.uk/article_details.php?id=7320

15 Keating F, Robertson D, McCulloch A, *et al*. Op. cit.

16 Ferns P. Op. cit.

17 Phillips T. Opening speech at the Race Convention 2006. Available at: www.cre.gov.uk/Default.aspx.LocID-0hgnew0nu.RefLocID-0hg00900c002.Lang-EN.htm

18 Cobain I. Inside the secret and sinister world of the BNP. *The Guardian*. 21 December 2006. Available at: www.guardian.co.uk/farright/story/0,,1976649,00.html

19 Ferns P. Op. cit.

20 Information Centre about Asylum and Refugees in the UK. *A brief history of refugee settlement in Leicester*. 2005. Available at: www.icar.org.uk/?lid=1050

21 Leicester City Council Social Care and Health Department. *The Annual Report of the Interpretation and Translation Service*. Leicester: Leicester City Council; 2005.

22 Subbuswamy K. *Analysis of assessments made under the Mental Health Act in Leicester in 2003*. Leicester City Council (unpublished internal report); May 2005.

23 Bartlett J. In: Ellix S. Briefing on the recommendations for action from the Department of Health report *Delivering Race Equality in Mental Health Care: an action plan for reform inside and outside services*, and the Government's response to the Independent Inquiry into the death of David Bennett. Leicester City Council Social Care and Health Department; July 2005.

24 Akwaaba Ayeh. *Annual Report 2005–2006*. Akwaaba Ayeh Mental Health Project. Leicester; 2006. Available at: akwaaba@akwaabaayeh.com

25 Patel N, Patel B (BP & Associates Ltd). *Research Project on Children and Adolescent Mental Health Service for Black and Minority Communities in Leicester and Leicestershire*. Leicester City Council (unpublished internal report). 2004. Available at: bpa.ltd@ntlworld.com

26 Leicester City Council Social Care and Health Department. Op. cit.

27 Wadsworth G. *Report on the cost effectiveness of the translating and interpreting service*. Unpublished internal report. Sure Start, Highfields. Leicester; October 2006. Available at: surestarthighfields-partner@nspcc.org.uk

28 Bartlett J. *Genesis: Annual progress report on the mental health consultation and planning support project for the city of Leicester*. Unpublished internal report. Leicestershire Action for Mental Health Project (LAMP). 2004. Available at: jamesbartlett@lampdirect.org.uk.

29 Shooter M. In: Partners in Care Campaign; 2005. Available at: www.rcpsych.ac.uk/campaigns/partnersincare/summary.aspx

30 Fernando S. Op. cit.

31 Department of Health. *Shift . . . Same World, Different View: action on stigma report into ending discrimination at work*. London: Department of Health; 2006. Available at: www.dh.gov.uk/assetRoot/04/13/95/69/04139569.pdf

32 MacAttram M. In: 1990 Trust/Black Information Link (website press release). 'Lord Patel resignation highlights disaster of government's mental health policy'; 15 December 2006. Available at: www.blink.org.uk/pdescription.asp?key=13522&grp=5

33 Sainsbury Centre for Mental Health. *Costs of Race Inequality*. London: Sainsbury Centre for Mental Health; 2006. Available at: www.scmh.org.uk/80256FBD004F3555/vWeb/flKHAL6UGM45/$file/costs_of_race_inequality_policy_paper_6.pdf

CHAPTER 6

Race and mental health: there is more to race than racism

SWARAN P SINGH and TOM BURNS

[This chapter is reproduced in full with permission from the BMJ Publishing Group. Originally published as an article in *BMJ* 2006; **333**: 648–51.]

Some minority ethnic groups in England and Wales have higher rates of admission for mental illness and more adverse pathways to care. Are the resulting accusations of institutional racism within psychiatry justified?

> It occurred to me that there was no difference between men, in intelligence or race, so profound as the difference between the sick and the well.
>
> F Scott Fitzgerald. *The Great Gatsby.* 1925

The 'Count me in' census for England and Wales showed higher rates of admission for mental illness and more adverse pathways to care for some black and minority ethnic groups and produced predictable accusations of institutional racism within psychiatry.[1] Lee Jasper, chair of African and Caribbean Mental Health, stated: 'This census confirms once and for all that mental health services are institutionally racist and overwhelmingly discriminatory. They are more about criminalising our community than caring for it.'[2] In fact, the census clearly states that it 'highlights the differences between various black and minority ethnic groups and the need to avoid generalisations about these groups. It does not show a failure in the services' (page 7) and comments that 'although many possible explanations have been put forward for these patterns, the evidence is inconclusive' (page 27). Not surprisingly it was the accusation of institutional racism, described as a 'festering abscess within the NHS,'[2] that made the headlines. Mr Jaspers is not alone in expressing such concerns. Several reports and inquiries have also alleged that psychiatry is institutionally racist.[3-6] What, then, is the evidence that the census findings can be attributed to racism within psychiatry?

RATES OF MENTAL ILLNESS IN MINORITY GROUPS

High rates of mental illness in migrant groups have been recognised and speculated on throughout the past century. A scientific approach to understanding the issue originated with Odegaard's observation of raised rates in Norwegian immigrants in Chicago,[7] and various theories have been proposed to explain excess.[8] In the United Kingdom the argument is at its most intense around the enduring epidemiological finding of high rates of psychosis in second generation African-Caribbean patients.

These higher rates have been proposed as evidence of racism on two main grounds. Firstly, that the diagnoses are mistaken, stemming from 'Eurocentric' diagnostic practices; Western psychiatrists are proposed to be more likely to misinterpret behaviour and distress that is culturally alien to them as psychosis. It is unfamiliarity with culturally alien ideas and practices that leads psychiatrists to label some black and ethnic minority people's behaviour as 'bizarre' or illogical (characteristics of psychotic psychopathology). In short, the patients neither have the illness nor the symptoms attributed to them but are simply misunderstood by intellectually rigid and inattentive professionals. The second argument is that even if the diagnosis is not that amiss the clinical response is powerfully influenced by racial stereotypes. It is argued that the compulsory detention of black patients, by itself, reflects entrenched discriminatory value judgments.

Contrary to the view that 'there has been little debate' and 'little inclination to address' racism within mental health services,[9] psychiatry is not complacent about these issues. Indeed, an impressive body of high quality research focuses explicitly on them. To date, no population group or culture has been identified in which psychotic disorders do not occur.[10] There are some variations in incidence and course of psychotic disorders across cultures, but what is striking is the similarity of phenomenology.[11-13] A diagnosis of psychosis is therefore not made because ethnic minority groups 'deviate from white norms' or on 'Eurocentric' theories or even in a 'futile search for "black schizophrenia".'[9,14,15]

A series of UK studies has been conducted specifically to test the theory that culturally derived misdiagnosis explains excess rates of psychosis in ethnic minority patients. Using highly structured and validated research diagnosis assessments by independent raters, these studies have consistently confirmed high rates of psychosis in the African-Caribbean population (particularly second generation immigrants) and also not found any raised rate of misdiagnosis.[16-18] The excess of psychosis in the African-Caribbean community in the UK is real and well accepted by epidemiologists and researchers.[8,19]

Rates of psychotic disorder are high not just among the African-Caribbean community in the UK, they are high for all immigrant groups globally.[20] The excess is also not restricted to non-Western minorities. Rates of schizophrenia are high in migrants to Denmark from Australia and Greenland,[20] in Finnish migrants to Sweden,[21] and in Britons, Germans, Poles, and Italians who migrated to Australia.[20] Increased rates of psychosis in all migrants, irrespective of ethnicity, therefore suggests an explanation that is not ethnic specific and is environmental rather than genetic. Shared experiences of discrimination, social exclusion, and urbanicity may all contribute to this increased risk and also explain a greater increase in communities exposed to higher levels of such experiences, such as black and ethnic minority communities in the UK.[20-22] Ethnicity and psychosis is simply not a black and white issue.

COMPULSORY DETENTION IN MINORITY GROUPS

High rates of detention and adverse pathways to psychiatric care for ethnic minority patients have been confirmed in many UK studies: racism within psychiatry and racial stereotyping of such patients are the commonest explanations provided for this excess, with little evidence to substantiate or refute this claim (Greenwood *et al.* 'Ethnicity and Mental Health Act 1983: a systematic review.' Submitted to the Department of Health 2006). A study by Lewis found that UK psychiatrists rated black male patients as potentially more violent than white patients.[23] However, a similar study by Minnis conducted 10 years later reported a contradictory finding – that UK psychiatrists were more likely to regard white patients as a management problem and to pose a risk of violence to others.[24]

A recent multicentre UK study of first episode psychosis, while confirming excess detention and more adverse pathways to care for African-Caribbean patients, also found lower rates of referral from general practitioners and higher referrals from the criminal justice system.[25,26] Intriguingly African-Caribbean families were more likely to access help for an ill family member through the police rather than the medical system. Since this was a study of presentation of first episode psychosis to secondary and tertiary services, this finding cannot reflect prior experience of institutional racism within psychiatry. The authors postulate that the greater stigma of mental illness in the African-Caribbean community might act as a barrier to early help seeking until a crisis develops, when the behavioural disturbance of the illness is misconstrued by families as requiring legal rather than medical help. The excess of detention rates is less striking for Asian than African-Caribbean patients and is lower in first episode psychosis than more chronic illness (Greenwood *et al.* 'Ethnicity and Mental Health Act 1983: a systematic review'). This strongly points towards important and as yet unexplored differences between ethnic minority groups in factors that contribute to detention. It also suggests that, over time, the relationship between ethnic minority patients and mental health services deteriorates, thereby creating a spiral of downwards engagement, in which each illness episode contributes to further disengagement and hence more coercive management strategies.

The decision to detain a patient is necessarily preceded by the patient's refusal to accept help on a voluntary basis. Hence, a legitimate question is whether some groups of patients are more likely to refuse help from psychiatric services. And if so, why? We know that individuals who have no intermediary (usually a family member) to help them access help are more likely to receive compulsory care, partly because carers may seek help early and pre-empt an acute crisis and partly because of fewer community alternatives to detention such as an extended family or support network. Other factors associated with higher detention rates – such as unemployment, living alone, low levels of social support, and non-compliance with medication – are higher in some ethnic minority groups.[27-29] Indian and Pakistani patients, while as socially deprived as African-Caribbean patients, are almost invariably brought to services (general practitioner or psychiatrist) by family members, which may explain why rates of compulsion among them are not as high as for African-Caribbeans.[30] Other important and as yet under-researched areas such as ethnic differences in help seeking and explanatory models of illness may further explain higher detention rates in some ethnic minority groups.

CONSEQUENCES OF ACCUSATIONS OF RACISM

These findings are quoted not to blame the victim but to highlight that there are perfectly reasonable alternative explanations for why the rates and manner of admission vary between different ethnic groups. Construing racism as the main explanation for the excess of detentions among ethnic minorities adds little to the debate and prevents the search for real causes of these differences. Alienation and distrust of the statutory services among inner-city black youth is not restricted to the mental health services. In psychiatry, accusations of racism simply feed into ethnic minority communities' alienation and mistrust of services. They create a self fulfilling prophecy whereby ethnic minority patients are primed to expect services to be poor and racist, decline all offers of voluntary admission, are detained, and disengage with services over time.

Institutional racism would hardly be a credible explanation for the excess of diabetes in South Asians in Britain or hypertension in African-Caribbeans. Why do we accept it so readily in mental health? The blunt use of the term racism perpetuates conceptual confusion and inhibits the search for more credible explanations.[31] It also leads to a series of damaging consequences for the profession, ethnic minority groups, and, most crucially, for ethnic minority patients.

The claim of institutional racism damages the profession and patients. Firstly, such a vague, meaningless yet insulting accusation contrasts with real attempts over the past 50 years to move away from mystifying jargon that cannot be interrogated. It devalues the thoughtful research that has been conducted to better understand these problems. It undermines morale and recruitment as staff feel undervalued and blamed. Secondly, it distracts both professionals and the minority communities from trying to understand these very real differences. Blaming others may bring temporary comfort but is hardly likely to lead to increased understanding and remedial action. Thirdly, and most gravely, it damages the welfare of current and potential ethnic minority patients. If they anticipate a racist and discriminatory reception from us, then it is no surprise that they stay away from needed help until it is too late and there are few alternatives to detention and enforced treatment.

GETTING BEYOND BLAME

Mental health practice has to build on trust. Trust can still be built, even when there are real differences of perspective. If these painful but legitimate differences are simply dismissed as racism then there is little ground for such trust and understanding to grow. Racism is indeed prevalent in society. It is deeply damaging to individuals and certainly contributes to the problems of ethnic minority communities. There are real ethnic inequalities in mental healthcare, which deserve closer attention and remedial action. It is likely that racism, combined with economic disadvantage and social exclusion, contributes to poor experience of psychiatric services for minority communities. This should be explored in methodologically sound, hypothesis driven research, not simply accepted as the global explanation for all ethnic differences in mental illness and healthcare.

There are several fruitful avenues for understanding ethnic inequalities and thereby improving services for ethnic minority patients. Ethnicity is a complex multifaceted concept, but insufficient attention has been given to the most appropriate methods of classification of ethnic group.[32] More research is needed that distinguishes between different ethnic groups. Longitudinal studies that monitor the development of therapeutic relationships between ethnic minority patients and services over time should help identify factors that influence detention rates – such as engagement, access, and appropriateness of services. Future research should also look in depth at the process of application of the Mental Health Act. The true denominator for such studies is the population assessed for detention, not just the sub-group that is detained. The differential rate of detention may indeed be a function of lesser availability of alternatives to hospital treatment in certain ethnic groups. Data relating to both assessment and detention should therefore be routinely and centrally collected.

It is also vitally important that detention is not seen as a punitive measure. The Mental Health Act is an enabling act; it allows services to ensure that treatment is available for those most in need of it. The decision to detain an individual under the Mental Health Act involves a complex interaction between clinical judgment, the patient's psychopathology, risk, fulfilment of legal requirements, local availability of resources, and the patient's refusal to accept help on a voluntary basis. Simplistic explanations of racism as the only determinant of such complex processes simply reinforce prejudices without offering any solutions. There is a serious risk to potential patient care if charges of institutional racism deter staff from taking clinically appropriate decisions and actions. The factors that contribute to excess detention even in the first episode of mental illness must operate before presentation to mental health services. Hence, any potential solutions must go beyond the health sector and involve statutory as well as voluntary and community agencies. The problem does not reside exclusively in psychiatry and hence the solutions cannot emerge from psychiatric services alone.

Summary points
The 'Count me in' census for England and Wales showed higher rates of admission for mental illness and more adverse pathways to care for some black and minority ethnic groups and led to accusations of institutional racism within psychiatry.
This accusation of racism as an explanation for these findings is erroneous, misleading and ultimately counterproductive.
It leads to several damaging consequences for the profession, ethnic minority groups, and, most crucially, for ethnic minority patients.
It acts like a self fulfilling prophecy by contributing to mistrust of services by ethnic minorities, thereby leading to delayed help seeking with increased use of detention and coercive treatments for ethnic minority patients.

REFERENCES

1 Commission for Healthcare Audit and Inspection. *Count me in. Results of a national census of inpatients in mental health hospitals and facilities in England and Wales.* London: Commission for Healthcare Audit and Inspection, 2005. www.healthcarecommission. org.uk/_db/_documents/04021830.pdf

2 MacAttram M. *Census reveals unprecedented levels of racism within the NHS.* 15 Dec 2005. National Black and Minority Ethnic Mental Health Network. www.bmementalhealth. org.uk/index.php?option=com_content&task=view&id=46&Itemid=1 (accessed 1 Aug 2006).

3 Department of Health. *Delivering race equality in mental health care: an action plan for reform inside and outside services and the government's response to the independent inquiry into the death of David Bennett.* London: DoH, 2005. www.dh.gov.uk/ assetRoot/04/10/07/75/04100775.pdf

4 *Independent inquiry into the death of David Bennett.* Cambridge: Norkolk, Suffolk and Cambridgeshire Strategic Health Authority; 2003. www.nscstha.nhs.uk/4856/11516/ David%20Bennett%20Inquiry.pdf

5 National Institute for Mental Health. *Inside outside. Improving mental health services for black and minority ethnic communities in England.* London: Department of Health; 2003. www.dh.gov.uk/assetRoot/04/01/94/52/04019452.pdf

6 *Breaking the circles of fear: a review of the relationship between mental health services and African and Caribbean communities.* London: Sainsbury Centre for Mental Health; 2002. www.scmh.org.uk/80256FBD004F6342/vWeb/pcPCHN6FMJWA

7 Odegaard O. Emigration and insanity. *Acta Psychiatr Neurol Scand Suppl.* 1932; **4**: 1–206.

8 Sharpley M, Hutchinson G, McKenzie K, Murray RM. Understanding the excess of psychosis among the African-Caribbean population in England: review of current hypotheses. *Br J Psychiatry Suppl.* 2001; **40**: s60–8.

9 Sashidharan S. Institutional racism in British psychiatry. *Psychiatr Bull.* 2001; **25**: 244–7.

10 Jablensky A. Epidemiology of schizophrenia. In: Gelder MG, Lopez-Ibor JJ, Andreasen N, editors. *New Oxford Textbook of Psychiatry*. Oxford: Oxford University Press; 2000: 592.

11 Jablensky A, Sartorius N, Cooper JE, Anker M, Korten A, Bertelsen A. Culture and schizophrenia. Criticisms of WHO studies are answered. *Br J Psychiatry*. 1994; **165**: 434–6.

12 Sartorius N, Jablensky A, Korten A, Ernberg G, Anker M, Cooper JE *et al*. Early manifestations and first-contract incidence of schizophrenia in different cultures. A preliminary report on the initial evaluation phase of the WHO Collaborative Study on determinants of outcome of severe mental disorders. *Psychol Med*. 1986; **16**: 909–28.

13 Srinivasa Murthy R, Kishore Kumar KV, Chisholm D, Thomas T, Sekar K, Chandrashekari CR. Community outreach for untreated schizophrenia in rural India: a follow-up study of symptoms, disability, family burden and costs. *Psychol Med*. 2005; **35**: 341–51.

14 Sashidharan SP, Francis E. Racism in psychiatry necessitates reappraisal of general procedures and Eurocentric theories. *BMJ*. 1999; **319**: 254.

15 Fernando S. *Mental Health, Race and Culture*. Basingstoke: Palgrave Macmillan; 2001.

16 Van Os J, Castle DJ, Takei N, Der G, Murray RM. Psychotic illness in ethnic minorities: clarification from the 1991 census. *Psychol Med*. 1996; **26**: 203–8.

17 King M, Coker E, Leavey G, Hoare A, Johnson-Sabine E. Incidence of psychotic illness in London: comparison of ethnic groups. *BMJ*. 1994; **309**: 1115–19.

18 Bhugra D, Leff J, Mallet R, Der G, Corridan B, Rudge S. Incidence and outcome of schizophrenia in whites, African-Caribbeans and Asians in London. *Psychol Med*. 1997; **27**: 791–8.

19 Bhugra D, Bhui K. African-Caribbeans and schizophrenia: contributing factors. *Advan Psychiatr Treat*. 2001; **7**: 283–91.

20 Cantor-Graae E, Selten JP. Schizophrenia and migration: a meta-analysis and review. *Am J Psychiatry*. 2005; **162**: 12–24.

21 Hjern A, Wicks S, Dalman C. Social adversity contributes to high morbidity in psychoses in immigrants: a national cohort study in two generations of Swedish residents. *Psychol Med*. 2004; **34**: 1025–33.

22 Wicks S, Hjern A, Gunnell D, Lewis G, Dalman C. Social adversity in childhood and the risk of developing psychosis: a national cohort study. *Am J Psychiatry*. 2005; **162**: 1652–7.

23 Lewis G, Croft-Jeffreys C, David A. Are British psychiatrists racist? *Br J Psychiatry*. 1990; **157**: 410–15.

24 Minnis H, McMillan A, Gillies M, Smith S. Racial stereotyping: survey of psychiatrists in the United Kingdom. *BMJ*. 2001; **323**: 905–6.

25 Morgan C, Mallett R, Hutchinson G, Bagalkote H, Morgan K, Fearon P *et al*. Pathways to care and ethnicity. 1: Sample characteristics and compulsory admission. Report from the AESOP study. *Br J Psychiatry*. 2005; **186**: 281–9.

26 Morgan C, Mallett R, Hutchinson G, Bagalkote H, Morgan K, Fearon P *et al*. Pathways to care and ethnicity. 2: Source of referral and help-seeking. Report from the AESOP study. *Br J Psychiatry*. 2005; **186**: 290–6.

27 Cole E, Leavey G, King M, Johnson-Sabine E, Hoare A. Pathways to care for patients with a first episode of psychosis. A comparison of ethnic groups. *Br J Psychiatry.* 1995; **167**: 770–6.

28 Burnett R, Mallett R, Bhugra D, Hutchinson G, Der G, Leff J. The first contact of patients with schizophrenia with psychiatric services: social factors and pathways to care in a multi-ethnic population. *Psychol Med.* 1999; **29**: 475–83.

29 Sellwood W, Tarrier N. Demographic factors associated with extreme non-compliance in schizophrenia. *Soc Psychiatry Psychiatr Epidermiol.* 1994; **29**: 172–7.

30 Koffman J, Fulop NJ, Pashley D, Coleman K. Ethnicity and use of acute psychiatric beds: one-day survey in north and south Thames region. *Br J Psychiatry.* 1997; **171**: 238–41.

31 Bhugra D, Bhui K. Racism in psychiatry: paradigm lost–paradigm regained. *Int Rev Psychiatry.* 1999; **11**: 236–43.

32 Singh SP. Ethnicity in psychiatric epidemiology: need for precision. *Br J Psychiatry.* 1997; **171**: 305–8.

CHAPTER 7

Child and adolescent mental health services in England

MICHAEL MAHER and CATHY STREET

SETTING THE SCENE

Child and Adolescent Mental Health Services (CAMHS) in England encompasses a wide range of services, arranged in a broad four-tier structure – spanning primary-level services at Tier 1 through to the most specialist (often inpatient) services at Tier 4. These multi-disciplinary services cover the age range 0–18 years and work with many different types of health needs, employing a variety of treatment approaches and increasingly work in non-health settings such as schools, alongside the more 'traditional' clinic settings found in the National Health Service (NHS).

This chapter does not set out to offer an overview of the state of CAMHS in England in 2007. This has already been done in two recent publications, which set out the progress which has been made over recent years.[1] Rather, the aim here is to set CAMHS in its current context, to outline some of the key issues facing CAMHS development and then to describe some of the organisational issues which beset the commissioner, manager and clinician in their attempts to work towards and within a comprehensive CAMHS.

These challenges are explored using a systems-centred perspective, with the authors drawing upon their quite contrasting experiences of working in the CAMHS field (one author (CS) is a researcher and consultant and the other (MM) has experience of instigating, planning and setting up a new multi-agency service) to make sense of the patterns observed.

DELIVERING CAMHS IN 2007: CLEARLY ON THE NATIONAL POLICY AGENDA

For many years in England, there were concerns that mental health services for children and young people were a 'Cinderella' service, with much greater attention being paid – and NHS budgets allocated – to adult mental health services. Likewise, a much higher profile was given to mental illness in adults in comparison with that afforded to children and adolescents.[2] This situation has changed dramatically over the last decade – partly because of a growing understanding of emotional and psychological development, but also because the wider and lasting implications the disorders than can affect young people became more widely recognised.[3] Giving further impetus to this shift, a number of influential reports were published, too, which highlighted that over the last 30 years, there has been a significant increase in mental health problems in children and young people.[4]

Nowadays, one of the most commonly quoted statistics is that one in 10 children or young people experiences some form of mental health disorder. The past three years have seen a belated recognition of this, with a serious investment in CAMHS. Following on from a *National Service Framework* (*NSF*) focused on the mental health of adults, the *National Service Framework for Children, Young People and Maternity Services* (often called 'the Children's *NSF*') was published in 2004 and, through a Public Service Agreement (PSA) target, requirements for a comprehensive service to be commissioned in all areas of England by the end of 2006 were set out.

There are multiple indicators for what so-called comprehensive CAMHS should include and cover, with 'proxy' measures which will mark the CAMHS impact on the wider system for children and young people, but it has been left to local contexts to decide on how best this should be configured. The three proxy measures – the short-term priorities – include access to 24-hour and emergency cover; services and transitional arrangements for young people (16- and 17-year-olds) and CAMHS services for children and young people with learning disabilities. Medium-term priorities include, amongst others, the development of: partnership working; early intervention and primary care; paediatric liaison; provision for looked-after children; routine outcome monitoring and evidence-based practice. Some of these will require considerable investment in the infrastructure and information technology/ information and data collection systems within CAMHS.

Running alongside these developments have been some more overarching challenges that apply to all NHS services, namely: the emergence of extensive guidance on commissioning services and a commissioning framework;[5] the emphasis on joint planning, commissioning and the pooling of budgets;[6] the requirements to develop service user participation and involvement;[7] and the emergence of Children's Trusts with an emphasis on collaborative working.[8] Also, specifically in relation to health services for young people in the mid-teens and early-20s, the emphasis has been placed on improving the interface between mental health services for children (CAMHS) and adult mental health services (AMHS) – another area of long-standing concern and where the recent government interest in social exclusion has played a key role.[9]

CHILDREN'S MENTAL HEALTH AS 'EVERYONE'S BUSINESS'

In many respects, all of the above might suggest that this is a time of considerable opportunity for CAMHS – a coming together of investment and recognition that children's mental health concerns everybody, especially all professionals associated with the well-being of children. Furthermore, it is too important and big a job for any one agency to be able to deliver the service needed to cater for the level of need of England's children in the 21st century.

It is also, then, a time of significant shift in service provision for CAMHS professionals, away from a traditional specialist service (although the need for specialisms obviously remains) to involvement in a wider system (or set of systems). Within the latter, CAMHS is a shared responsibility, and the CAMHS professional's job involves both discharging his or her clinical specialism directly with patients, and acting as a resource inside the system to help others to address mental health needs in the way they go about their jobs. Thus CAMHS becomes twin track – a specialist service and a connected part of universal services for children. This move takes it from a service which is appropriate for a discrete, relatively small group of children to potential involvement in shaping the cultural context for the development of all children. The justification for this shift comes from the prevalence of mental illness and mental health problems in children and young people, as noted earlier.

The evidence points to some real improvements in CAMHS over the past five years:[10]

➤ expenditure on CAMHS rose from £284 million in 2002–03 to an estimated £513 million in 2005–06, an increase of over 80%
➤ an increase in CAMHS staffing occurred over the period 2003–05 of 2115 whole-time equivalents, equal to 27%
➤ CAMHS saw more cases – an increase in total caseload of 32 382 cases from 2002 to 2005 (40%) and an increase in new cases of 21 508 (219%).

At the same time, it is clear that there is anxiety about the fragile nature of some of the improvements, and the need to overcome some significant challenges in a number of areas if improvement is to be built upon. We will return to the anxiety later. For example, the report just cited, which detailed the progress made towards meeting the *NSF*, also noted:

> a significant proportion of children who could benefit are still not receiving services. Research has shown that only 25 per cent of children with a diagnosed psychiatric disorder were accessing mental health services over a three year period.

As well as the *NSF*, the other main driver for change has been the Every Child Matters: Change for Children programme, which is led by the Department for Education and Skills to ensure that every child has the appropriate levels of support that he or she needs to:
➤ be healthy
➤ stay safe
➤ enjoy and achieve
➤ make a positive contribution
➤ achieve economic well-being.

The two initiatives obviously overlap – indeed the *NSF* can be seen as 'nested within' the ECM programme – and all CAMHS activity is to be measured and reported on under both domains.

A chapter of this length cannot go any further into the detail of the complexity of the current context of CAMHS, or deal with all the dimensions noted so far. A recent report summed up the state of things:

> the context within which comprehensive provision for child and adolescent mental health can be established is immensely complex and totally dependent upon a whole-systems approach to joined-up service planning, delivery and evaluation.[11]

SYSTEMIC FACTORS IN A CHANGING CONTEXT

In the rest of this chapter we will concentrate on what factors contribute to the likeliness of success of a whole-systems, partnership-based approach, and what factors militate against the potential for success. With such an approach, CAMHS has a chance of successfully meeting the expectations which accompany the investment in it; without it, any progress will be fitful, temporary and unsustained. In order to clarify our thinking, we will use a systemic approach to the understanding of group and organisational change and development.[12]

From this perspective, systems survive, develop and transform via the discrimination and integration of difference. Difference in this context is synonymous with information flow across the boundary. Boundaries close and become impermeable when a system reacts to what is perceived as too much difference – this can also be called a defensive retreat into the familiar. For systems to come out of such retreats and engage with the reality of the context – the changing context – they have to be able to work on integrating the new, the unfamiliar, the different. If they are successful in this, they will begin to reform their defensive positions – the system will begin to see similarities in the apparently different, and differences in the apparently similar. From this position it is possible for the boundary to become appropriately permeable again, not too closed so that new and important data are kept out; not too open so that members of the system feel swamped and overwhelmed with the undifferentiated enormity of it all. Then it becomes possible to think about what might need to happen – how we might need to change what we do – so that we can ensure that we are acting in synchrony with the wider system's priorities.

As well as too much difference, the other factor that causes a system boundary to close is 'noise' in the system, here defined as ambiguity, confusion and redundancy. These factors are experienced as static in a radio transmission – it becomes hard to understand what information is being conveyed and listeners shut their ears to the discordancy.

In a nutshell, the theoretical framework above gives us a template to apply to the experience of CAMHS teams undergoing or facing profound change. What factors might be required for the changes to be engaged with creatively, with enthusiasm and buy-in? What factors might be present which will act as restraining forces to the success of the enterprise?

PARTNERSHIP, LEADERSHIP AND CHANGE

We have already noted that a whole-systems approach is necessary to the delivery of a comprehensive service, and strong and effective partnerships are key to this. The central partnership groupings have to struggle with the issues outlined above – if they can survive, develop and transform, then the various service changes they are leading have a chance to create a niche in which they can operate. Such groupings operate across local authority and Primary Care Trust (PCT) groupings as CAMHS strategy groups or the like. What challenges do they face and how can they thrive?

The first challenge is that of the difference of cultural background. Such groups need to include and involve managers and clinicians from Health, Social Care, Education and other partnership agencies. On its own, this can prove a barrier which has been underestimated – the sense of difference can be too much for the group to integrate and it can become unproductive and stale, as illustrated by the following:

> When they work, partnerships establish a structure that brings clarity and support to all; but endless energy can be squandered trying to bring different players together in ineffective groups. Partnerships may be fragile and often need to be nurtured; support from specialist consultants in organisational psychology/group relations can be extremely helpful.[13]

This foundation group needs to develop beyond its early phase of development in which cultural differences are experienced to the exclusion of similarities. This can be experienced as a kind of deafness to what actually is going on – the internal dynamic arranges itself along lines of stereotype sub-grouping – 'I agree with you because I am on your side; I disagree with you because you belong to a different grouping, and I always disagree with them.' Such stereotyping along lines of organisational affiliation, professional grouping or core training runs deep and most groups deal with it by pretending it is not there.

In such cases, flight and fight impulses are acted out in endless debates in seemingly rational terms. The tenor of these discussions often goes along a pattern of proposal – 'Yes, but . . . (opinion) . . .', 'Yes, but . . .', 'Yes, but . . .', 'Yes, but . . .'[14] Let us give an imaginary dialogue to illustrate this.

A I think we should set aside some time to really define the role of Primary Mental Health Workers.

B Yes, but they actually cover a number of different roles, depending on where they are in the system.

C I think they are already too disparate, and their roles do need to be defined more clearly.

D But it's actually quite valuable to have different strengths and skills to call upon, depending on what the situation requires.

A Yes, but they are all paid on quite a high grade, and there are some real differences in expertise and skill.

E Yes, but that should have been addressed when the job profiles were first developed and the recruitment was done – I did ask everyone for input then and I got nothing back . . .

This group is behaving as if it is on task, but a quick review of the communication patterns reveals the opposite. Each speaker is joining the discussion on a difference – the 'Yes, but' tag is a way of pretending an agreement which is actually a contradiction. It is as if there can be no building on one another's views, ideas, experiences and thoughts, not to mention feelings. The underlying dynamic is that of fight – the covert group task is to spend its energy on fighting. The chance of anything productive coming out of the meeting is correspondingly low, and the blame for the group's being bogged down and not making things happen will be put down to other people's being awkward.

The above scenario is common enough in any context – it is all the more likely to apply when change is experienced as overwhelming and where there are multiple differences to be managed. In the CAMHS context, we have a significant change to the system as a whole and, at the same time, the constituent parts – particularly PCTs and local authority Social Service and Education departments – have been going through and continue to undergo radical changes. Under these conditions, there are many reasons to get stuck like the group we have described.

So systems such as this are in danger of closing to too much difference, and becoming bogged down in fight. What about the other factor, that of 'noise' in the system? Here again, the great difficulty of bringing together already large and structurally complex organisations into larger even more structurally complex organisations can threaten the improvements in functioning that it is designed to facilitate. Challenges include:

➤ ambiguity – CAMHS have to work in partnership, but uncertainty is rife about how to join up, with whom, to do what, for which outcomes[15]

➤ contradictions – one agency's priority target may not be another agency's interest, yet they have to work together (the most striking example of this lies between the domains of Health and Education, where priorities and targets commonly point in very different directions)

➤ redundant duplication – CAMHS will be subjected to multiple external assessments, providing data via many different plans and monitoring processes. Where multi-agency services exist, they may be inspected both by Ofsted and the Health inspection agency, and the results can sometimes be contradictory.

So we have twin dangers – too much difference, and too much noise. What such systems need, then, is help to clarify what their top priorities are, and help to filter out noise in the system, and help to get the group working to see similarities – common issues, problems, areas of potential opportunities to avoid duplication – the fact that the children and the problems they bring are common to everyone. The most important factor in giving and sustaining this help is that of leadership, in the form of people in key positions who can act as champions for CAMHS across services, and who can hold a vision and keep momentum going in service development. Where this leadership has been consistent and supported, so that there is enough clout at a high enough level across the organisations involved to unblock stoppages in the system and sort out system problems, then these are the contexts in which partnership working has got off the ground and proved productive.

The obvious danger to this dependency on leadership is the amount of change going on in all the partner organisations, such that the figures who are key to service development and who sustain the momentum will themselves move on, voluntarily or not. It is at these times that the ground which has been made feels most fragile, and this may partly account for the sense of anxiety often expressed about the gains that have been made.

THE EXPERIENCE IN PRACTICE

An example may be useful here. One local authority wanted to develop services with CAMHS which would be part of the answer to the performance indicator:

> Were protocols in place for your council area for partnership working between agencies for children and young people with complex, persistent and severe behavioural disorders?

The process for beginning to think about ways of working with the group defined (loosely) in the above question took six years. It was six years before a service started up, and it has taken a further two years before that service can be described as fully functioning and effective. During that time, the local authority Social Services and Education departments merged to form a Children's Service, and the three PCTs which covered the area were disbanded and amalgamated into one. All the constituent organisations also had significant reorganisations which resulted in very high levels of staff turnover.

The initial thinking began with a steering group, a sub-group of the CAMHS strategy group, made up of personnel from the three PCTs (clinicians and managers), the Education department and Social Services. This group struggled with the basic concept of shifting preoccupation away from diagnostic categories and institutionally driven responses with the concomitant question of treatability, and onto a different way of approaching complexity and young people in crisis.

The traditional questions – those of inter-sectoral territorialism – were:

'What is the diagnosis? To whom, then, does this child "belong"? Who is going to pay for his or her care/treatment?'

(Clearly there is a pressure here for the questions to be answered in such a way that the answer will be 'not us'.)

The questions the group aimed to shift it to were:

'What is the nature of the crisis? What intervention could we make to reduce the crisis? What sets of skills would be needed to effect such an intervention, and in what context?'

It took years of repeated effort for this group to engage with planning a service which could begin to provide answers to these questions, and all the time the struggle was to avoid slipping back into the old questions. Behind the struggle there were anxieties in the wider system – some saw it as a secret takeover of Health by Children's Services, and clinicians who became involved and supportive of the plan were attacked for collaborating and 'selling out'. In Children's Services, anxieties abounded about Health's using the opportunity to screen out referrals, and not really engaging with the hardest-to-reach clients.

These issues notwithstanding, the service development continued to make progress, supported by the strategy group and its management of the pooled budget. That it made such progress rested on there being enough key players remaining in the agencies who identified with the aspirations it represented, and who understood enough about its increasingly labyrinthine structural foundations in terms of budgets, staffing, managerial processes and the rest. There were enough such people – just about – but it was touch and go. By the time the service started, two out of the original group remained in post. Two years on, none of the originating group remains. Others have taken on the identification and ownership, and the signs are that the service has had the start it needs to move from survival into development and transformation, but it is easy to see from this successful example how easy it is for complex initiatives to founder.

The significant word in the foregoing story is 'complex', but perhaps this is misleading, and 'complicated' might be a more accurate term. It is well recognised that for producing complex products or outcomes, you need simple structures. It is also well known that there is a danger that often the opposite happens, and complicated structures are built, with the task of producing complex outcomes or products. Financial and managerial processes in the NHS are famously Byzantine in their obscurity and cumbersomeness; those of local authorities aspire to match them in these qualities. When combined, there quickly develops a situation which is so confused and 'noisy' that it threatens to bury the fragile emerging newborn under the weight of its own complicated mess.

LESSONS

The driving belief behind the development of the service described above was that of the need for professionals to come together to treat, educate and care for young people with needs that went beyond the boundaries of any single agency. The drive towards such wider system integrations has been enshrined in the *NSF* and in Every Child Matters, but the energy and resilience required to overcome the resistance represented by too much difference and too much noise seems to have been dangerously underestimated.

In their foreword to the recent report into progress towards implementation of the *NSF*, the governmental 'parents' of the reforms acknowledge:

> The NHS is going through a period of unprecedented change . . . In the short term the structural changes which underpin this system reform may pose challenges for some CAMHS.[16]

Our concern is that in this understatement lies a huge amount of frustration and some despair. In the example given it was not possible to create a simple structure – all the existing organisational processes militated against this. So a service was constructed with staff from four separate employers, with different terms and conditions and different policies and procedures governing their employment. The financial underpinning was too complicated for any one person to have a full understanding – and this is before any clinical complexity is engaged in, and before the service attempted to influence any embedded behaviours in the wider system. In effect, the service was born before the context was ready for it. The parent system had not developed the organisational structures in which such a service could develop in a way which was structurally simple, to leave the way clear for engaging on complex clinical pioneering work. As a result, much of the energy, ingenuity, resilience and creativity which could have gone into developing effective ways of working with young people whose needs had outstripped other single-agency attempts to work with them went instead into trying to get the host systems to accommodate themselves to the newborn and to give it the support it needed to survive.

It is our argument that the foregoing is, in microcosm, representative of the critical challenge to developing a genuinely comprehensive CAMHS service. Too much energy has gone into developing over-complicated systems which struggle to work effectively; for CAMHS to meet the challenges facing it, there will need to be the political and organisational courage to simplify structures and organisational processes, so that energy can be directed towards necessarily complex work with complex clients. A first critical milestone has passed in terms of the proxy targets for CAMHS – that of 31 December 2006. We must also remember, however, that this is only the beginning of a 10-year journey. Sustaining the progress made to date, and maintaining momentum, will require the ongoing attention of all working in this demanding field.

REFERENCES

1 Department of Health, Department of Education and Skills. *Promoting the Mental Health and Psychological Well-being of Children and Young People.* Report on the Implementation of Standard 9 of the National Service Framework for Children, Young People and Maternity Services. London: Department for Education and Skills, Department of Health; 2006.
  Kurtz Z, Lavis P, Miller L, *et al. Developing Comprehensive CAMHS.* London: Young Minds; 2006.
2 Audit Commission. *Children in Mind.* London: Audit Commission; 1999.
3 Ibid.
4 Rutter M, Smith DJ, editors. *Psychosocial Disorders in Young People: time trends and their causes.* Chichester: John Wiley; 1995.
5 Department of Health. *Health Reform in England: update and commissioning framework.* London: Department of Health; 2006.
  Department of Health. *Review of Commissioning Arrangements for Specialised Services.* London: Department of Health; 2006.
6 Department of Health. *Joint Planning and Commissioning Framework for Children, Young People and Maternity Services.* London: Department of Health; 2006.
7 Department of Health. *Patient and Public Involvement in Health: the evidence for policy implementation.* London: Department of Health; 2006.
8 University of East Anglia. *Children's Trusts: developing integrated services for children in England.* London: Department for Educations and Skills; 2005.
9 Social Exclusion Unit. *Transitions: young adults with complex needs.* London: Office of the Deputy Prime Minister; 2005.
10 Department of Health, Department of Education and Skills. Op. cit.
11 Kurtz Z *et al.* Op. cit. p. 21.
12 Agazarian YM. *Systems-centered Therapy for Groups.* New York: Guilford; 1997.
13 Kurtz Z *et al.* Op. cit. p. 15.
14 Simon A, Agazarian YM. SAVI: the system for analyzing verbal interaction. In: Beck AP, Lewis CM, editors. *The Process of Group Psychotherapy: systems for analyzing change.* Washington, DC: American Psychological Assn; 2000. pp. 357–80.
15 Kurtz Z *et al.* Op. cit. p. 23.
16 Department of Health, Department of Education and Skills. Op. cit. p. 4.

CHAPTER 8

Third age mental health services: all our tomorrows?

JONATHAN HILL and GERALD O'MAHONY

CONTEXT

At a recent social gathering the first topic of conversation amongst a group of middle-aged males was not the price of property, the problems of educating their high school-/university-age children nor even global warming and the environment – it was concerns about the ongoing independence of their parents and their ambivalence about gently prompting their parents into a 'care home'. Unaware that they had a 'specialist' in their midst, they were genuinely seeking support and advice from each other – the conversation lasted some time and it transpired that each one was wrestling or had wrestled with these questions over their own parents.

Having spent many years in a speciality which has never been glamorous, thrilling or terribly technical, it is suddenly quite surprising to us to find that what has always been a Cinderella subject is now becoming of interest to a very wide section of the population. Why should this be?

AN AGEING POPULATION

It has become a truism that we are living longer and healthier lives and, just as the benefits are being celebrated, the problems that this causes are becoming recognised. The pensions funding gap, with the prospect of a rising retirement age, and the concerns about the proportion of working-age people to those of retirement age are two, but by far the most pressing is the rapid expansion of the 'very' old. Even without the ageism implicit in that category, people are living longer and healthier after they retire but then they may also enter a longer period of ill-health in their senescence before they die.

Thus, although the incidence of diseases affecting the extremes of old age is not changing – for example, Alzheimer's disease affects perhaps 1% of 65-year-olds, 10% of 75-year-olds, 20% of 85-year-olds – the huge growth in the number of people moving into their ninth or tenth decade means that the prevalence of such illnesses is growing exponentially. Thus at a conservative estimate of a 2% annual growth in the susceptible population over 20 years, there will be a 50% increase in prevalence of Alzheimer's in that time span.

If services are to catch up and then keep pace with demand, it will be essential for decision-makers and those setting priorities to recognise the changing nature of the future needs of an ageing population. This generation has a vested interest in getting our services right – if providing services for our parents, the 'war' generation, is already a challenge, then how much more difficult is it likely to get when the next 'baby boomers' generation reach old age?

BIOTECHNOLOGY

Research into all aspects of ageing, but particularly the ageing brain, is burgeoning, generating new possibilities for diagnosis and management. We may look forward to the advent of advances in prevention and treatment if not cure, but these are likely to be complex and multi-factorial and not the silver bullet of popular mythology. Increased understanding of the role of nutrition, lifestyle and assorted health risks in the aetiology of mental health problems in the elderly will lead to individual's being able to make healthier choices to reduce their likelihood of developing problems later in life.

Increasing demands will be felt for non-invasive forms of investigation, such as imaging, with a range of more sophisticated and costly structural and functional scanning techniques being seen as routine procedures.

Should the promise be realised of new forms of treatment becoming available, particularly drugs which could alter the course of Alzheimer's disease, this would inevitably and naturally result in a huge increase in demand for rapid screening along the lines of the two-week rule for cancer assessments. While this might ameliorate or, for many, solve the problem of the burden of long-term care, it would entail a huge shift in resources towards early diagnosis in mild or minimal cognitive impairment and for the provision of expensive treatments for those affected.

CONSUMERISM

Expectations about quality and levels of care have risen progressively since the National Health Service (NHS) was founded almost 60 years ago. This is seen in all fields of medicine, so for example it is now not questioned that an 80-year-old with renal failure should receive dialysis if they are physically fit in other respects. Rising national wealth combined with a rising proportion of that wealth being spent on health through the NHS have addressed these demands, but there remain significant pressure points particularly in mental health services for the third age.

Current and future generations of sufferers and carers ('consumers of healthcare') have been raised with the expectation of treatment by the NHS and there is a 'multiplier' effect of people (partners, children and their partners) whose lives are being affected by these illnesses. A further catalyst to their demand would be clearer evidence that such treatment (whether the acetyl cholinesterase inhibitors or others) delayed or avoided the need for residential care and so delayed the moral, emotional and financial crisis accompanying such a decision.

In addition, there are increasing expectations of choice enshrined in the language of autonomy and supported by the Human Rights Act and the Mental Capacity Act. Inevitably the majority of constraints to choice are due to restricted resources (whether financial or skills/people based) – those who are wealthy enough can afford to fund their choices but for the majority, there will always be a degree of rationing of resources. Historically it has been the articulate middle classes who were able to exercise choice within the statutory sector and it remains a challenge to service providers to ensure that services are needs based rather than demand led.

RESOURCES

Paradoxically, as financial resources in the NHS have grown, the availability of long-stay, NHS-provided beds for people (mostly elderly and mostly with dementia) has declined dramatically. This reduction was initially more than matched by a dramatic expansion in private nursing and residential beds funded liberally by Health and Social Services. As standards have been raised and public costs curtailed, many of the smaller homes have been forced to close leaving only the larger commercially profitable homes to survive.

Despite this, the move to community care has everywhere been welcomed – particularly when it results in imaginative and co-operative solutions for people with chronic illness being able to remain in their own home.

However, there remains the problem of recruiting enough carers to provide the care. The same demographic changes which result in an altered balance between the working/retired population also result in a shortage of working-age carers who can be employed to support care in the community. The growth in the number of extremely old (i.e. over 90) people results in many of their children having to act as carers, when they themselves are in their 70s, or even their spouses who are likely to also be of advanced age. Just as the supermarkets and other large employers are beginning to recognise the value of their knowledge, skills and dedication, it is likely that the social services and non-statutory care agencies will need to start recruiting from the elderly population itself.

On the assumption that the chronic effects of ageing cannot be avoided, there will also arise the issue of residential home or nursing-home care when care in the community becomes 'unviable'. Currently this largely equates to its cost-effectiveness, i.e. if the home-care package is more expensive than residential or nursing-home care, then it will not be funded by the statutory sector. In the future, support may be rationed by the availability of carers. Further constraints occur in the 'real' world, with recent evidence suggesting that the number of residents necessary for an independent home to remain financially viable is inexorably rising. So, far from the small 'home away from home' image that the independent sector tries to project, we are in danger of falling into the 'institutional care' trap levelled for so many years at NHS-provided long-term care.

Resource pressures generated by the demands of older people and their carers have been highlighted by the controversy over the National Institute for Health and Clinical Excellence (NICE) guidelines regarding acetyl cholinesterase inhibitors. The Institute initially gave a qualified green light to the prescription of these drugs, while the 2001 guidelines implicitly rationed their prescription by recommending that it was limited to 'specialists' after full multi-disciplinary assessment. This was not on the grounds of risk, as these drugs have been well trialled in the elderly and are not particularly hazardous.

A review was promised and, when the outcome of this review appeared likely to result in the withdrawal of this group of drugs from NHS prescription (i.e. not from the market but from the list of drugs that the NHS considered as cost effective and would pay for), there was an outcry. A great deal of public pressure was put on NICE to enter into consultation, with a view to altering its recommendation. NICE, however, works to explicit criteria which are set down by the Government and as such took the opprobrium for what was in essence a political decision about financial priorities.

MODELS OF HEALTHCARE

The elderly have always figured large in the traditional medical model of healthcare, if only because the majority of non-infectious diseases occur with increasing frequency with advancing age, whether this is chronic debilitating illness such as arthritis or the onset of terminal illness. The original retirement age of 65 was pragmatically set because most manual workers were no longer fit to work beyond this age; those working in the 'old' professions of the law, the clergy and medicine had greater liberty to go on working beyond this age.

This no longer holds true and the retirement age is now more flexibly set at somewhere between 65 and 75, with further adjustments in the statutory retirement age being proposed. Within the Social Services context, an 'older adult' is now someone over 50 whilst the NHS still retains a cut-off age of 65 for its 'geriatric' services. Anti-age discrimination legislation will inevitably alter this, but there will still be the need for targeting and specialisation to deal with the complex social, psychological and physical needs of older adults.

As the average age of the population has increased and each generation's length of time in retirement can be expected to be significantly greater than the preceding generation's, what defines old age has to be reassessed. The co-existence of a number of acute and chronic illnesses in one individual (multiple pathology) is a particular characteristic of this group and a generation of generalist physicians came to be trained as 'geriatricians' in order to deal with the complexities of treating such patients, supporting them back into independent living through rehabilitation programmes. The move towards greater sub-specialisation, both in the medical and surgical fields, has meant that older people increasingly receive their care from those sub-specialists after direct referral from their own general practitioner, providing protection from any discrimination based around criteria based solely on age. The geriatrician is increasingly expected, as a hospital-based physician, to be involved in the emergency care of non-elderly patients and to carry out procedures that might not be part of their routine work with the elderly, perhaps at the cost of failing to perfect their skills of caring for the older patient. The debate continues as to whether the elderly are best supported by generic or specialist services.

Dedicated mental health services for the elderly are relatively recent, evolving over the past 25 years. Though these developments have been increasingly supported by the NHS, the services have largely been driven forward locally by pioneering clinicians. The marginalisation of older people's mental health in the context of national developments of mental health strategy or within older people's health provision is so consistent throughout all levels of planning that it appears to represent an unconscious form of institutional ageism. The recent developments of *National Service Frameworks* (*NSFs*)[1,2] for both mental health and older people's health have led to rising expectations. The development of a comprehensive mental health service for old age was only touched upon by both. The faultlines opening between systems and structures allow older people's provision to slip out of sight – the profile of the elderly within mental health being low and the position of older people's mental health failing to achieve priority in any over-arching health policy for the aged. The fact that this is usually unrecognised and, when highlighted, denied, does not rescue the situation from the double jeopardy where the category of mental health is not acknowledged as part of the older person's agenda nor is the needs set of the older person adequately attended to when considering developments in mental health services.

INTEGRATION

There has also been a gradual realisation that meeting the healthcare needs of the elderly is not only the preserve of medical services but is best approached through joint working between Health and Social Services and across both statutory and voluntary agencies providing a network of care.[3] Requirements are for a whole-systems methodology with shared planning designed to meet a range of needs across housing, welfare benefits provision, health promotion and work aimed at protecting the vulnerable adult and engaging the older citizen in continuing to seek access to educational and recreational activities. Increasing emphasis is being placed upon joint working across agencies and voluntary-sector organisations. Health-funded bodies are being given the freedom to purchase social care through changes in the law pertaining to the spending of NHS funds – so-called Section 31 Agreements – and through health and social care statutory agencies commissioning work through the voluntary sector, such as occurs with the development of advocacy services provided by the Alzheimer's Society or the mental health charity, MIND.

THE CARE ENVIRONMENT

Some 65% of people with dementia are cared for at home[4] and the overwhelming majority of people with long-term functional mental illness (depression, schizophrenia and so on) are not hospitalised, the latter receiving similar packages of care to their counterparts of working age. For many, the later stages of illness will still demand entry into institutional care.

The process of closure of large psychiatric hospitals has been balanced by the increasing number of privately provided and sometimes publicly purchased beds. There is an inherent tension in the system that varies between means-tested Social Services funding with an NHS 'contribution' for any nursing component and funding from the NHS which is free at the point of delivery and even prevents top-up funding for additional elements of care. This conflict is unresolved but has been actively debated in the media and is still subject to legal challenge and ultimately to political decision-making.

In parallel with this relative disinvestment in care for the elderly, there is an increasing focus on the public safety agenda of targeting those with mental illness who are perceived to be threatening to society, the so-called 'forensicisation' of mental health. Much of the additional spending on mental health that has occurred in the past few years has gone into providing high-quality care for offenders with mental health problems. Whether provided through NHS hospitals, private hospitals or nursing home facilities, such services by their very nature tend to exclude older adults; indeed the presence of a dementing illness appears to prevent patients from accessing these necessarily expensive facilities.

The proposed remodelling of mental health legislation to encompass the category of dangerous personality disorder is in itself redefining the role and scope of psychiatry, so that it will be become even less focused on the elderly, frail and other dependent groups.

THE LEGAL FRAMEWORK

Only recently has the legal system begun to address the specific mental health problems of vulnerable groups as opposed to those who were perceived as threatening to society. The long-awaited Mental Capacity Act addresses many of the specific problems of the elderly and of people with learning disability. It aims to facilitate clearer decision-making around health and welfare issues, protecting the vulnerable elderly as well as promoting their autonomy. It will enable an individual to make specific advance decisions and also permits substitute decision-making for the first time.

The Act will require Mental Health Trusts and Social Service departments to formulate policies around its principles. This will result in much more explicit decision-making and greater transparency but undoubtedly also in an increase in detection/recognition of mental health problems in the elderly.

In the future, the Mental Capacity Act will ensure that all those persons who lack capacity to make a decision (in this context, usually relating to whether to enter residential care) or who are held in *de facto* detention (whether in hospital or in a community setting) will be offered specific legal protection. In the case of people with no relative or friend to act in their interests, this will be through the appointment of a statutory independent mental capacity advocate. For the first time it will also become a specific criminal offence to ill-treat or neglect someone who lacks capacity – and for carers there will be statutory protection when acting to meet the needs of an incapacitated adult.

SERVICE DELIVERY

Traditionally services were hospital based and dominated by the delivery of care through inpatient beds separating the organically ill (largely dementia) from the functionally ill (such as those with depression or schizophrenia). Day hospitals were seen as a link between the hospital and the community to support independent living and to provide assessment and treatment instead of a hospital admission or to facilitate earlier hospital discharge.

Currently favoured models of service centre on a community-based service with the provision of local Mental Health Teams for older adults. The blueprint is of a multi-disciplinary and multi-agency service acknowledging that positive mental health requires the maintenance of community ties and a network of support systems that is constructed by fostering communication between the statutory and voluntary sectors as well as across Health and Social Services, such that an elderly person encountering problems will be identified earlier and may expect an appropriate response. Implicit in this model is the expectation that early intervention will promote health maintenance rather than commit high-cost resources to meet the needs of those with established ill-health. History teaches that the development of a proactive service itself will generate increasing volumes of work as previously unrecognised health needs are brought to light. Many of the antecedents of psychological ill-health remain embedded in a complex matrix of social and economic realities. When planning for service development, strategists increasingly have to base projections on census data and what is known of local demography.

Much has been done to benchmark older people's mental health services against national standards, allowing local services to measure their range of provision and state of development. It is hoped that the development of performance indicators will allow commissioning bodies to ensure value is obtained for public expenditure.

There is a debate as to whether older people should have access to the full range of services that are available to adults of working age, such as 24-hour home treatment or Assertive Outreach Teams. Arguments range over whether the provision of such resources is simply a manifestation of equitable service delivery or whether it is a prescriptive model representing a disproportionate commitment of resources from what are often small, specialised teams where developing services might prefer the flexibility of exploring models of service that are tailored to local circumstances.

SPECIALIST SERVICES

The growth of our population of older citizens has required both the development of specific services but equally a recognition that the range of demands being made necessitates new ways of working. Particular attention has been given to early intervention and assessment for the conditions prevalent in old age. Strategies for the management of long-term health conditions are being promoted both in primary and secondary care. Attempts are being made to deliver care closer to home and, for those who are admitted, provision is being made to allow for early supported discharge. Partnerships are being developed to try to respond to the needs being expressed by older people and their families.[5] The promotion of initiatives identifying best practice and attempts to encourage named staff to take on the role of champions of older people's needs have been features of recent developments.

A range of themes has been considered by relevant bodies, work to agree upon standard-setting has been undertaken by collaboration between professional groups such as the Royal Colleges of Psychiatrists and Physicians,[6] endorsed by the voluntary sector and the Government's Care Services Improvement Partnership (CSIP). The starting point is to promote health as far as is possible by providing for interventions at community and primary care level. Following on, defining the multi-disciplinary skill set that should be in place to constitute an adequately equipped community Mental Health Team for older adults is critical. Similarly, training for Health and Social Care workers is seen as a priority, as it encourages the recognition of treatable mental health problems such as depression which, though prevalent, all too often go unrecognised.[7] Memory Assessment Services to assist in the recognition and detection of dementia are being promoted, with services being set up to meet newly established norms for protocols around investigation and management.[8]

The provision of psychological therapies for those in late life has been something commonly omitted in service planning and is now identified as a central feature of an adequate service for the elderly. The capacity of a local service to introduce such support is seen as a measure of the commitment that a given service has to putting aside barriers to accessing healthcare on grounds of age.

INTERFACE ISSUES

That the older person may require the involvement of services from across the spectrum of Health and Social Care sets its own demands. It is necessary to establish ways of collaborative working that facilitate transfers of information without duplication. This sets new challenges around information management technology, promoting information exchange that respects confidentiality by working within constraints laid down by data protection legislation.

As individuals negotiate healthcare pathways between services, the need to have agreed policies for the transfer of care becomes increasingly important. Without such policies, particular groups are at risk of being left behind – such as those with learning difficulties, those with dementia of young onset or isolated groups such as elderly prisoners.

It is necessary to develop psychiatric services that are alert to the needs of older people entering general hospitals. At any one time, two-thirds of hospital inpatients will be aged 65 and over and it is estimated that perhaps one in three elderly patients may become acutely confused during such periods of hospital care,[9] requiring the establishment of liaison psychiatric services linking the Mental Health Team to acute hospital services.

The capacity of the service to avoid unnecessary inpatient care or promote early discharge to the home will depend upon the flexibility of whole systems working across Health and Social Care partnerships. The introduction of intermediate care or step-down units is necessary to facilitate the transition from a period of acute dependency in an inpatient setting. Such care is more akin to a residential placement supported by staff with a range of therapy skills, including the occupational therapist or physiotherapist. Services are required to agree protocols ensuring that those with mental health needs will have access to the full range of such provision and this remains one of the central tasks of strategic planners for those with the responsibility for commissioning services.

CONCLUSION

As a rising tide will lift all boats, spending increases in real terms over a decade have seen improvements work their way through into mental health services for older people. Developments in social policy promoting joint working between all relevant parties have given rise to a feeling of optimism that services for the elderly can continue to become more effective. The pace of change promoted by government-driven health initiatives has to an extent marginalised developments in older people's mental health as the public safety agenda, more often associated with the Home Office than the Department of

Health, has taken centre stage. There appears to be a movement to commit the Government to the development of an integrated set of guidance initiatives to promote the improvement of mental healthcare in the elderly.[10,11] However, the sheer volume of guidance taken with the increasingly prescriptive nature of policy changes working in a command economy model threatens to overload the abilities of staff to adapt to potential change.[12] Although the delivery of improved services may be within our grasp, increased demand will equate to unmet needs so long as resource limitations are in place. While a high profile is given to public involvement in setting priorities for healthcare,[13] the conflicting needs of a growing group of ageing citizens against a proportionally smaller group charged with funding Health and Social Care predicts that areas of tension will continue to emerge over many years to come.

REFERENCES

1 Department of Health. *National Service Framework for Mental Health.* London: Department of Health; 1999.
2 Department of Health. *National Service Framework for Older People.* London: Department of Health; 2001.
3 Care Services Improvement Partnership. *Everybody's Business: integrated mental health services for older adults – a service development guide.* London: Department of Health; 2005.
4 Dementia UK. *Summary of Key Findings.* London: Alzheimer's Society; 2007.
5 Audit Commission. *Forget-Me-Not: mental health services for older people.* London: Audit Commission; 2000.
6 Royal College of Psychiatrists. *Raising the Standard: specialist services for older people with mental illness.* London: Royal College of Psychiatrists; 2006.
7 National Institute for Clinical Excellence (NICE). *Depression: management of depression in primary and secondary care.* NICE Clinical Guideline 23. London: NICE; 2004.
8 National Institute for Health and Clinical Excellence. *Dementia.* NICE Clinical Guideline 42. London: NICE; 2006.
9 Clinical Effectiveness and Evaluation Unit, Royal College of Physicians. *The Prevention, Diagnosis and Management of Delirium in Older People.* Concise Guidance to Good Practice No. 6. London: British Geriatrics Society; 2006.
10 Care Services Improvement Partnership. Op. cit.
11 Philp I, Appleby L. *Securing Better Mental Health for Older Adults.* London: Department of Health; 2005.
12 Hall J, Waldock H, Harvey C. Improving mental health services for older people. *Ment Health Rev.* 2006; **11**(4): 7–13.
13 Warburton D. *Evaluation of Your Health: your care, your say.* London: Department of Health; 2006.

CHAPTER 9

Services for depression, anxiety and post-traumatic stress disorder

JONATHAN I BISSON

Depressive disorders, anxiety disorders and post-traumatic stress disorder (PTSD) account for around 70% of all psychiatric disorders found in the general population.[1] They usually result in distress for the sufferer and those around them and are associated with functional impairment. In addition to the personal cost of these disorders, the cost to society is immense. Murray and Lopez[2] have estimated that the global burden of unipolar major depression will be second only to ischaemic heart disease by 2020.

Thankfully several effective treatments are available for depression, anxiety and PTSD, and it is vital that sufferers are aware of them and can access appropriate services that provide them. Unfortunately there remain big gaps in awareness and service provision that need to be addressed. In recent years many secondary mental health services have focused their resources on individuals who suffer from 'serious and enduring mental health difficulties'. A proportion of sufferers of depression, anxiety and PTSD would be considered to fall into this category but many would not, leaving providers and sufferers concerned that their needs are not appropriately catered for.

In the last three years the National Institute for Health and Clinical Excellence (NICE) has performed exhaustive systematic reviews of the literature and synthesised the information gathered from them regarding the management of depression, anxiety and PTSD. This has led to the publication of three comprehensive guidelines on their management[3-5] (all available to download from: www.nice.org.uk). These documents not only summarise the current evidence but also provide guidance against which local NHS organisations should review their management of clinical conditions. It is hoped that

NHS providers will adopt the NICE guidelines in a timely manner and that these guidelines will underpin current service provision and inform it in the future.

In this chapter the three disorders are defined and the key management recommendations of the NICE guidelines described. This is followed by consideration of service provision at present and how it could be developed in the future.

DEPRESSION

The characteristic features of a depressive episode include depressed mood, loss of interest and enjoyment, reduced energy leading to increased fatigue and diminished activity, reduced concentration and attention, reduced self-esteem and self-confidence, ideas of guilt and unworthiness, bleak and pessimistic views of the future, ideas or acts of self-harm or suicide, disturbed sleep and diminished appetite.[6] Three grades of severity are used: mild, moderate and severe. The severe form of depression is sub-divided into severe depressive episode without psychotic symptoms and severe depressive episode with psychotic symptoms, where an individual has delusions, hallucinations or depressive stupor in addition. Sadly, for many, depressive episodes recur, leading to a diagnosis of recurrent depressive disorder. Some individuals also experience elation of mood and are classified as having a bipolar (manic depressive) disorder. This chapter focuses on individuals with depressive episodes or recurrent depressive disorder, as opposed to bipolar disorder.

The replication of the United States National Co-morbidity Survey[7] found that 16.2% of the United States population had suffered from a diagnosable depression at some time in their life, with 6.6% of the population suffering from a depressive disorder in the preceding 12 months. Of those who had a depressive disorder in the preceding 12 months, 10.4% were classified as mild, 38.6% as moderate, 38% as severe and 12.9% as very severe. The mean episode duration was found to be 16 weeks, although for a significant proportion the length of episode was much longer.

Depression affects individuals of all ages. There is a very similar ratio of males to females and several factors have been associated with an increased risk of depression, including stressful life events and genetic factors (there is good evidence that depression can run in families). Other factors that have been associated with depression include having several young children, unemployment and economic difficulties. There is also an increased rate of depression amongst those with physical disorders.

Management of depression

The NICE guidelines for depression[8] note the heterogeneous nature of depression and the fact that different management approaches are likely to be beneficial for different people, depending on the presentation. A particularly important point for depression sufferers, indeed for all individuals presenting with mental health difficulties, is that the effective assessment and subsequent co-ordination of care may significantly contribute to improved outcomes. A comprehensive assessment should consider the psychological, social, cultural and physical characteristics of the individual and the quality of their interpersonal relationships. The synthesis of this assessment should lead to the development of an appropriate management (or care) plan that is based on an individual's specific needs. Research has shown that several different treatment approaches may be equally effective for particular presentations of depression. In such instance an individual's preference and the experience and outcome of previous treatments should help to determine the approach to adopt. The NICE guidelines recommend a stepped care model, with roles for both primary and secondary care (Figure 9.1).

- Recognition of depression in primary care and general hospital settings.

- Management of recognised mild depression in primary care.

- Management of recognised moderate to severe depression in primary care.

- Involvement of specialist mental health services including crisis teams for treatment-resistant, recurrent, atypical and psychotic depression and those at significant risk.

- Depression needing inpatient care.

FIGURE 9.1 Stepped care model for the management of depression.

The stepped care approach

The majority of individuals with depression will present to their general practitioner (GP) and never come into contact with secondary mental health services. It is therefore vital that primary care professionals are able to successfully detect and manage depression. Depression sufferers may require care at any of the levels described below. Those who require more intensive care will usually require less intensive care once improved. For the majority of depression sufferers who require input from primary care or secondary mental health services, this will be time limited – although a significant minority will receive longer-term input.

Mild depression

For mild depression there is better evidence for non-pharmacological approaches than for pharmacological approaches. The NICE guidance suggests the following general measures: sleep and anxiety management; watchful waiting (following an initial assessment and discussion with a healthcare professional, the mild depression sufferer would be reviewed around two weeks later); exercise; guided self-help (this often involves reading appropriate materials with some time-limited support from a healthcare professional) based on cognitive behavioural therapy (CBT). Brief problem-solving therapy, CBT and counselling of six to eight sessions are specific psychological treatments that have been shown to be effective in the treatment of mild depression. However, randomised controlled trials suggest that anti-depressants have little clinically important effect in mild depression and they are therefore not recommended as a first-line treatment. Anti-depressants do have a role as a second-line treatment for mild depression and when depression is associated with psychosocial or medical problems, or when sufferers have experienced more severe episodes of depression previously.

Moderate and severe depression

As the severity of depression increases, so do the risks to the individual and to others. An appropriate risk assessment is very important. It should never be forgotten that around 10% of people with a diagnosis of severe depression die of suicide. For moderate and severe depression there is much better evidence for the effectiveness of anti-depressant drugs. They appear to be as effective as psychological treatments and are more widely available. It is therefore recommended that in moderate depression, anti-depressant medication is routinely offered to all patients before psychological intervention and, if effective, continued for a routine period of six months. Ideally, however, a strong argument can be made for offering moderate depression sufferers a choice of a pharmacological or psychological approach in the first instance. Various anti-depressants have been shown to be effective, although selective serotonin re-uptake inhibitors such as citalopram and sertraline have been recommended as the most appropriate drugs for first-line use as they are less likely to be discontinued because of side effects. Of the psychological interventions, CBT and interpersonal therapy have the best evidence of efficacy for moderate to severe depression. The duration of treatment should be longer than for mild depression and is usually in the range of 16–20 sessions over six to nine months. There is less evidence for psychodynamic psychotherapy, although the NICE guidelines recommend that it may be considered for the treatment of the complex co-morbidities that may be present along with depression. Individuals who have met the criteria for depression for at least two years (i.e. suffer from chronic depression) should be offered a combination of CBT and anti-depressant medication.

Specialist mental health services

The point at which specialist mental health services are involved varies greatly. Local service configuration, usual practice of the GP, severity of illness, level of risk and availability of alternatives to secondary care are all key factors that determine when an individual is referred. Ideally the key factors would include severity, treatment resistance, recurrent presentations, atypical presentations, psychotic symptoms and significant risk. Many of the treatment approaches adopted are similar to those described above. Psychological treatment is often delivered by more experienced therapists and alternative drug treatments, higher-dose drug treatment and combinations of drug treatments are often used. Many depression sufferers in contact with mental health services also receive other input from a multi-disciplinary team including occupational therapists, social workers and community psychiatric nurses. In severe forms of depression, crisis resolution and home treatment may be used.

Inpatient care

This is usually reserved for individuals who are assessed as being at high risk of self-harm or suicide. In such instances the inpatient setting represents a place of safety and protection, allowing close observation to reduce risk if necessary. Medication and psychological approaches are often used but if adequate trials of treatment are ineffective or the condition is considered to be potentially life-threatening, electro-convulsive therapy is sometimes used for severe symptoms.

ANXIETY

Anxiety disorders are divided into phobic anxiety disorders, including agoraphobia; social phobias and specific phobias; and other anxiety disorders, including panic disorder and generalised anxiety disorder.[9] It is more common for individuals to present with a combination of anxiety and depression rather than with either one on their own. Many individuals who are diagnosed as suffering from a depressive episode have significant features of anxiety as well and some have a co-morbid anxiety disorder in addition to a depressive episode. Sometimes it is impossible to separate a combination of mild depressive and anxiety symptoms leading to a diagnosis of mixed anxiety and depressive disorder. During a comprehensive assessment, it often becomes apparent which symptom dominates the clinical picture and treatment usually focuses on this in the first instance. However, in some individuals it is very difficult to state that one is more problematic than the other. Fortunately, many of the treatments used have both anti-depressant and anxiolytic effects.

The main difference between phobic anxiety disorders and other anxiety disorders is that in the former, the anxiety is evoked only or predominantly by certain well-defined situations or objects. For example, in agoraphobia the anxiety is provoked by leaving home. Sufferers of agoraphobia commonly complain of becoming acutely anxious if they enter shops, are in crowds or travel alone. Specific phobias include a specific fear of heights, spiders or flying. With a specific phobia, fear is caused by the presence or anticipation of a specific object or situation and hence that situation is avoided, or endured with intense anxiety or distress. Conversely, panic disorder is characterised by recurrent attacks of severe anxiety (panic) that are not restricted to any particular situation or set of circumstances and are therefore unpredictable. In generalised anxiety disorder, the anxiety is generalised and persistent. Characteristic symptoms of anxiety include intense fear or discomfort, often accompanied by symptoms characteristic of a panic attack, i.e. palpitations, sweating, shaking, shortness of breath, feeling of choking, chest pain, nausea, dizziness, and a fear of losing control.

In the replication of the United States National Co-morbidity Survey,[10] the lifetime prevalence of panic disorder was 4.7%, agoraphobia without panic 1.4%, specific phobia 12.5%, social phobia 12.1% and generalised anxiety disorder 5.7%. Various factors are associated with the development of anxiety disorders. Genetic factors are again important, individuals with more anxious personalities are more likely to develop them and stressful life events can precipitate anxiety disorders. They often run a chronic course and without treatment the majority of sufferers continue to have their anxiety for two years or more.

Management of anxiety

A range of different management approaches have been advocated for anxiety disorders. These have been systematically reviewed leading to the publication of NICE guidelines on the management of anxiety[11] which, like the NICE guidelines for depression, recommend a stepped care approach (Figure 9.2).

As suggested by the stepped care model, the majority of management of anxiety disorders will take place in primary care as opposed to secondary mental healthcare and therefore the successful management of anxiety disorders relies heavily on primary care practitioners being able to competently and accurately assess anxiety sufferers and on appropriate treatments being available.

- Recognition and diagnosis.

- Treatment in primary care.

- Review and consideration of alternative treatments.

- Review and referral to specialist mental health services.

- Care in specialist mental health services.

FIGURE 9.2 Stepped care model for the management of anxiety disorders.

Specific treatments

For panic disorder, it is recommended that benzodiazepines, such as diazepam, are not prescribed as they are associated with a less good outcome. CBT, delivered for between seven and 14 hours over a maximum period of four months, has the best evidence for sustained improvement. The selective serotonin re-uptake inhibitors (which are recommended as a first-line treatment) and tricyclic anti-depressants have also been shown to be effective treatments along with self-help, particularly guided self-help. There is some emerging evidence that CBT delivered via a computer interface may be of value. If an individual has not improved with one of the above treatments, it is recommended that an alternative form be tried. If there is still no improvement, then referral to specialist mental health services is recommended where a thorough reassessment should occur. Options for further care include CBT with a more experienced therapist, treatment of co-morbid conditions, structured problem-solving, full exploration of pharmacotherapy and day support. For generalised anxiety disorder, benzodiazepines should only be used acutely. For longer-term benefits, the interventions with evidence for the longest duration of effect are CBT over 16–20 hours, anti-depressant medication, in particular selective serotonin re-uptake inhibitors, and self-help. Specific phobias are not covered by the NICE guidelines but also often respond well to CBT.

POST-TRAUMATIC STRESS DISORDER

Post-traumatic stress disorder (PTSD) is characterised by recurrent distressing re-experiencing (e.g. nightmares, intensive images following reminders), avoidance of reminders, numbing of general responsiveness and hyper-arousal (e.g. increased irritability and hyper-vigilance). It is precipitated by experience of an extreme traumatic event that evoked intense fear, helplessness or horror at the time.[12] The lifetime prevalence has been estimated at 6.8%[13] and the 12-month prevalence at 3.5%,[14] with around one-third suffering from a severe form of the condition. Co-morbidity is very common, especially with depressive disorders, panic disorder, other anxiety disorders and substance misuse or dependence. The factors most associated with the development of PTSD are the intensity of the trauma, perceived lack of social support and peri-traumatic dissociation.[15,16] Around 50% of PTSD sufferers will recover within two years of the diagnosis, but over one-third of individuals develop a chronic form of PTSD that persists six years after it developed.[17]

Management of PTSD

Prevention and early intervention

The NICE guidelines for the treatment of PTSD found no early intervention targeted at everyone involved in traumatic events to be effective. In fact, there is a suggestion that some individuals do worse with a specific intervention, individual psychological debriefing, than with no intervention at all. The NICE guidelines for early intervention are to offer immediate practical, social and emotional support; not to debrief individuals; and to consider acute symptomatic pharmacological management, e.g. for extreme sleeping difficulties. There is good evidence that trauma-focused CBT can reduce acute PTSD between one and three months after a traumatic event, leading to NICE's recommending this and giving consideration to developing systems to screen for individuals at high risk.

Chronic PTSD (present for three or more months)

Both psychological and pharmacological treatments have been found to help chronic PTSD. The systematic review performed by NICE found that psychological treatments focusing on the traumatic event appeared to be more effective than those that focused elsewhere and more effective than pharmacological treatments. This led to recommendations that that all PTSD sufferers should be offered a course of trauma-focused CBT or eye movement desensitisation and reprocessing, normally on an individual outpatient basis, usually for between eight and 12 sessions but more often following multiple traumatic events and if there is co-morbidity or traumatic bereavement. If there is little or no improvement, an alternative trauma-focused treatment or augmentation with pharmacological treatment should be considered. NICE recommended paroxetine or mirtazapine as drugs for first-line use in secondary care, with amitriptyline and phenelzine being reserved for secondary care use. Medication may also be used before trauma-focused psychological treatment as a result of PTSD sufferer choice, serious ongoing threat and, sadly, lack of availability of psychological treatment.

SERVICE PROVISION FOR DEPRESSION, ANXIETY AND PTSD

At present many individuals with clinically significant anxiety, depression and PTSD will not present to primary care, secondary care or non-statutory services and either live with their symptoms or use alternative measures to try to deal with them. Unfortunately this can lead to problems. For example, alcohol is often used to self-medicate in all three conditions.

There are several excellent examples in primary care of services being structured to deliver effective interventions for sufferers of these conditions, but, sadly, this is not always the case. Increasingly, general practices have counsellors attached to them who are able to provide brief therapies and will usually provide the initial psychological interventions. These are often helpful and many primary care counsellors do use evidence-based interventions, though not all do. Another stumbling block has been the fact that many counsellors are contracted not to take on individuals for more than six one-hour sessions, which falls short of the time recommended for all the interventions described above, except for brief work for mild depression. It is likely that for more individuals to be effectively treated in primary care – which for those with milder forms of the disorders (i.e. the majority of sufferers) is the most appropriate place to receive treatment – counsellors and other psychological therapists will need to be able to provide input for up to 16 hours per individual. It is important that in the future the therapies provided in primary care are the evidence-based ones that have been shown to be effective and not any watered-down ones, unless there is evidence that this does not diminish their effectiveness.

There remains a shortfall of adequately trained psychological therapists in primary and secondary care to provide appropriately for sufferers of anxiety, depression and PTSD. This is well recognised and led to the Labour Party's promising an expansion of psychological therapists in their manifesto for the last General Election. Lord Layard[18] has estimated a need for 10 000 extra psychological therapists, particularly with CBT skills, and recommended that they work from psychological treatment centres in dedicated buildings. Pilot psychological treatment centres are now being developed and evaluated in Newham and Doncaster. (*See* companion volume, *Mental Health Services Today and Tomorrow Part 1: experiences of providing and receiving care*, Chapter 4, for a more detailed description.)

At present it is likely that most individuals who present to primary care with depression, anxiety or PTSD will be offered medication. At times this is entirely appropriate but often it is prescribed first line instead of being reserved as a second-line intervention. The probable excessive initial prescription of medication for all three conditions is associated with the shortage of psychological therapists, but also with limited dissemination and adoption of NICE guidelines. This is a complex issue and not easy to solve. NICE has developed various strategies to improve implementation, but research suggests that guidelines and educational strategies on their own are unlikely to be effective. Gilbody and colleagues'[19] systematic review of studies in this area concluded that complex interventions were more effective than simple ones. Useful factors included combinations of clinician education, nurse case management and greater integration between primary care and specialist mental health services.

In secondary mental health services, most community mental health teams are not well equipped to deliver the NICE recommendations, particularly in a timely manner. Shortage of staff and lack of staff with appropriate skills appear to be two of the key issues associated with this. In order to be more time-effective, anxiety management has traditionally been offered to many anxiety sufferers in a group setting, but the evidence is limited for this type of intervention and individual work has a better evidence base. There are several other examples of sufferers being provided with less effective or apparently ineffective interventions due to limited availability of the gold standard of treatment. In the future, skill levels amongst staff should reflect the evidence base and prevent individuals being taken on for support only for prolonged periods whilst awaiting the appropriate psychological treatment that, in many areas, can take up to a year or more to be provided.

Clearly, major training and staffing issues have been alluded to above. Lord Layard[20] argues that an increase in the number of psychological therapists by 10 000 is feasible over a seven-year period, but this will require considerable investment. In the meantime, there are examples of relatively simple interventions that can improve capacity without requiring major new resources. For example, an innovative approach has been adopted in Cardiff to increase the number of psychological therapists available to treat PTSD. Existing mental health professionals and counsellors have been trained and supervised in the provision of trauma-focused CBT. This has resulted in the ability to provide more PTSD sufferers with evidence-based treatments and to provide the therapists with new skills that they can use in their day-to-day practice, often with community mental health teams.[21] In addition to increasing the available number of therapists, there is a need for further research to develop effective briefer management strategies and hence to increase capacity. For example, guided self-help and computer-based interventions have provided some promising initial results and are associated with the requirement of less resource.

This chapter has focused on the provision of specific treatments but the successful management of many sufferers of depression, anxiety and PTSD – especially those with more chronic or complex difficulties – relies upon input from other statutory and non-statutory agencies. There are many different agencies involved in providing care, and effective multi-agency, interdisciplinary working is required. Agencies should not be working in competition or opposition but in a joined-up manner that allows a common pathway of care to be developed that all agencies are signed up to. Social factors can play a major role in the development and maintenance of all three disorders. Issues such as (un)employment, housing and finances are often critical and need to be addressed in tandem with specific treatments. Many primary care and mental health services have developed positive working relationships with agencies such as JobCentrePlus, Housing departments and associations, the Citizens Advice Bureau and Social Services to address these issues. The non-statutory sector is also very important in providing such input. National charities such as MIND, the Shaw Trust, Combat Stress and many others provide significant input. Some evidence-based psychological interventions are provided by the non-statutory sector, although probably their main provision is of support, advice, advocacy and opportunities to engage with other initiatives that may complement treatment. The level of services provided varies from quite intensive support (e.g. day centre provision) to less intensive support (e.g. self-help groups and advice on where and how to seek appropriate support). Such services are vital but at present not always optimally linked with statutory services, leading to duplication or even inconsistent provision of input. In areas where the relationships between all providers of mental healthcare have been addressed, more comprehensive seamless services can be provided.

In order to translate the evidence base into practice, there is clearly a need to provide education to a range of different people. The general population needs to be able to recognise when its members are suffering from a treatable condition, and to know what help is available and how to obtain it. This could be helped by mass publicity and figureheads, such as celebrities, publicising the key issues to raise the profile of depression, anxiety and PTSD. Useful guidance for the general public is already available. For example, all three of the NICE guidelines discussed have produced publications aimed at potential service users that detail the recommendations and are designed to empower sufferers to obtain the interventions they require. One way of improving the situation in the future is to disseminate such information in a more effective manner. Increased pressure from users to receive the most appropriate levels of care is likely to be a powerful means of encouraging the changes in service configuration and spending that will be needed to provide optimal care. In addition to the public, providers need to be aware of the current evidence base. NICE has produced guidance specifically for GPs but improved dissemination of such guidance to all providers is required.

There remains a need for more specialist mental health services but, in the future, they are likely to continue to be restricted to taking on individuals with more complex difficulties or individuals who have not responded to first-line treatments. Configuration of services using a stepped care model should facilitate this and result in individuals being seen by the appropriate person or team for their individual needs. One concern about a purely stepped care approach is that individuals with more severe difficulties who are unlikely to respond to the initial steps are not seen by secondary services soon enough. To combat this, a more stratified approach should be adopted, whereby the initial assessment determines what level of care an individual needs and they receive this straight away. This is perhaps most apparent in the NICE guidelines for depression, where individuals with a severe depressive disorder would be offered different forms of intervention from those with milder forms of the disorder.

CONCLUSION

Service provision for depression, anxiety and PTSD is not optimal at present. The availability of effective treatments for all these conditions and pointers as to how services can be improved should lead to the development of more appropriately configured services with the capacity to effectively treat more people in the future.

REFERENCES

1 Kessler RC, Berglund P, Demler O, *et al*. Lifetime prevalence and age-of-onset distributions of DSM-IV disorders in the national comorbidity survey replication. *Arch Gen Psychiatry*. 2005; **62**: 593–602.

2 Murray CJ, Lopez AD. Alternative projections of mortality and disability by cause 1990–2020: global burden of disease study. *Lancet.* 1997; **349**(9064): 1498–504.

3 National Collaborating Centre for Mental Health (NCCMH). *Depression: management of depression in primary and secondary care – NICE guidance.* London and Leicester: Gaskell and BPS; 2004.

4 National Collaborating Centre for Mental Health (NCCMH). *Anxiety: management of anxiety (panic disorder, with or without agoraphobia, and generalised anxiety disorder) in adults in primary, secondary and community care.* London: NICE; 2004.

5 National Collaborating Centre for Mental Health (NCCMH). *Post-traumatic Stress Disorder: The management of PTSD in adults and children in primary and secondary care.* London and Leicester: Gaskell and BPS; 2005.

6 World Health Organization. *The ICD-10 Classification of Mental and Behavioural Disorders: clinical descriptions and diagnostic guidelines.* Geneva: World Health Organization; 1992.

7 Kessler RC, Berglund P, Demler O, *et al.* The epidemiology of major depressive disorder. Results from the national comorbidity survey replication. *JAMA.* 2003; **289**: 3095–105.

8 National Collaborating Centre for Mental Health (NCCMH). *Depression* . . . 2004. Op. cit.

9 World Health Organization. Op. cit.

10 Kessler RC, Berglund P, Demler O, *et al.* 2005. Op. cit.

11 National Collaborating Centre for Mental Health (NCCMH). *Anxiety* . . . 2004. Op. cit.

12 Kessler RC, Chiu WT, Demler O, *et al.* Prevalence, severity and comorbidity of 12-month DSM-IV disorders in the national comorbidity survey replication. *Arch Gen Psychiatry.* 2005; **62**: 617–27.

13 Kessler RC, Berglund P, Demler O, *et al.* 2005. Op. cit.

14 American Psychiatric Association. *Diagnostic and Statistical Manual of Mental Disorders (DSM-IV).* 4th ed. Washington, DC: American Psychiatric Association; 1994.

15 Brewin CR, Andrews B, Valentine JD. Meta-analysis of risk factors for posttraumatic stress disorder in trauma-exposed adults. *J Consult Clin Psychol.* 2000; **68**(7): 48–66.

16 Ozer EJ, Best SR, Lipsey TL, *et al.* Predictors of post-traumatic stress disorder and symptoms in adults: a meta-analysis. *Psychol Bull.* 2003; **129**: 52–73.

17 Kessler RC, Sonnega A, Bromet E, *et al.* Posttraumatic stress disorder in the National Comorbidity Survey. *Arch Gen Psychiatry.* 1995; **52**: 1048–60.

18 Layard R. *The Case for Psychological Treatment Centres;* 2006. Available at: http://cep. lse.ac.uk/layard/psych_treatment_centres.pdf

19 Gilbody S, Whitty P, Grimshaw J, *et al.* Educational and organisational interventions to improve the management of depression in primary care: a systematic review. *JAMA.* 2003; **289**(3): 145–50.

20 Layard R. Op. cit.

21 Kitchiner NJ, Bisson JI, Phillips B, *et al.* Increasing access to trauma focused cognitive behavioural therapy for post traumatic stress disorder through a pilot feasibility study of group clinical supervision model. *Cogn Behav Ther.* 2007; **35**: 251–4.

CHAPTER 10

Mental health, employment and housing

SARAH HILL, SIMON FRANCIS and ZOË ROBINSON

Access to employment and good-quality accommodation are key factors in determining an individual's life chances. People with mental health problems are particularly vulnerable and, relative to the rest of the population, are more likely to experience poor-quality housing and barriers to employment. This often results in an ongoing cycle of deprivation and exclusion that is all too often passed on from generation to generation. Employment is extremely important in maintaining mental health and promoting the recovery and well-being of those who have experienced mental health problems, as well as improving the quality of life. Stable, appropriate housing is critical as an underpinning factor contributing to the extent to which people feel able to progress toward work, and indeed to take an active part in community life. Mental health services, often in a pivotal position, have a crucial role to play in enabling people with severe mental health conditions to gain and retain employment and to access mainstream opportunities.

MENTAL HEALTH, WORK AND EMPLOYMENT

Article 23 of the United Nations' *Declaration of Human Rights* (1998) states that 'everyone has a right to work, to free choice of employment, to just and favourable conditions of work and to protection against unemployment'. Unemployment is allied to a decrease in general health,[1] and there is a strong relationship between unemployment and the development of mental health problems,[2] with an increased risk of suicide, predominantly amongst men under 35 years of age.[3,4] Work is therefore good for people.[5,6]

DEFINITIONS

Traditional definitions of work describe it as an activity that involves the exercise of skills and judgement taking place within set limits prescribed by others.[7] With the exception of some instances of self-employment, work is therefore essentially something you 'do' for other people. Employment is work for which people receive a regular wage whilst volunteering is unpaid work. If you are a 'worker', the National Minimum Wage applies and it has a legal standing and depends on the existence of a contract, implied or written.

THE ISSUES AND BARRIERS

People with severe mental health problems have the lowest employment rate for any of the main groups of disabled people. In England, the *Labour Force Survey* (2004) shows that 79% of people with mental health problems are unemployed whilst the situation is even worse for people with mental illness, who experience worklessness at a rate of 89%,[8] and now form the largest group of benefit claimants. Furthermore, the number of Incapacity Benefit claimants with mental health problems is nearly twice that of the previous decade.[9] However, many people with mental health problems want to work,[10,11] i.e. to be engaged in some kind of valued activity that uses their skills and meets the expectations of others.

The Social Exclusion Unit (SEU)[12] reported on the significant barriers that people can experience, including:
- ➤ low confidence due to the impact of mental health problems as well as the side effects from some medication
- ➤ low expectations among staff and a lack of knowledge about benefits and an over-cautious approach
- ➤ employer attitudes, often with the added hurdle of the Occupational Health Department's screening process
- ➤ difficulties moving from benefits to work, which can include lack of knowledge of the system, fear of having benefits unnecessarily cut and the financial implications of leaving benefits.

The report further identified the underlying causes of the social exclusion experienced by people with mental health problems, which include:
- ➤ stigma and discrimination, actual or fear of rejection from the community, which leads to people wanting to stay in the safety of mental health services rather than engaging in the mainstream
- ➤ a lack of clear responsibility between agencies for improving vocational and social outcomes for adults with mental health problems

➤ different services not always working effectively together to meet individual needs and maximise the impact of available resources

➤ diagnosis of mental health problems being missed or inaccurate, and a focus on medical symptoms rather than social and vocational roles

➤ professionals not having the time, training or local constraints to help people move into work or participate in their local communities

➤ fears about leaving benefits

➤ employers not knowing where to go for help.

Many of these issues are well rehearsed, and have since been confirmed during the National Social Inclusion Programme consultation for the Welfare to Work Green Paper *A New Deal for Welfare*, in 2006.[13] It is therefore important that, as a minimum, healthcare professionals are able to identify the key social issues that impact on an individual's employment and life chances, and where possible that they seek solutions. It is also important to keep in touch with ongoing policy developments, including those outside of the health system, in order to be able to give accurate information.

POLICY DEVELOPMENTS

There have been a number of recent policy and legislative developments from the Government, including welfare reforms and the drive to promote social inclusion, that indicate the importance of supporting people with mental health problems to obtain and retain work. Most recently the White Paper, *Our Health, Our Care, Our Say*[14] focuses on prevention, public health and well-being and a requirement to tackle inequalities and the support needs of people with long-term conditions. It emphasises the required support for people to return to work and accessing such schemes as Pathways to Work. The National Institute for Health and Clinical Excellence (NICE) also states that supported employment should be made available to people with schizophrenia, should they wish to work. The Cabinet Office's *Reaching Out: an action plan on social exclusion*[15] details the barriers faced by the most seriously excluded individuals and supports the Individual Placement and Support approach (IPS) in helping people with severe mental health problems return to employment, and in addition calls for a strategic regional response to this agenda. The Department of Health (DH) published *Vocational Services for People with Severe Mental Health Problems: commissioning guidance*,[16] which gives commissioners of mental health services a clear framework to deliver evidence-based vocational services for people with severe mental health problems and the tools to monitor the effectiveness of such services.

Welfare benefits are a fundamental aspect of social inclusion and directly link to employment and housing. The *Mental Health and Social Exclusion*[17] report highlighted benefit issues as an important perceived barrier to employment. The SEU's consultations highlighted that current rules are poorly understood and people believe that they would be worse off in work or hold perceptions that the job might not work out and therefore that they might need to reclaim benefits, which many suggested was difficult. In 2006, the Government implemented a series of changes to help address these challenges:

➤ Incapacity Benefit Linking Rules were made more flexible to allow people to return to the same level of Incapacity Benefit if they are unable to sustain a job because of their mental health
➤ abolition of benefit downrating occurred, which means that people in hospital for more than a year will keep receiving the same level of benefits that they had when they were originally admitted to hospital
➤ the Permitted Work Rules let people retain their benefits while working up to 16 hours per week, provided that their earnings stay within fixed limits
➤ the Working Tax Credit tops up the incomes of people on low wages working for 16 or more hours per week.

To further address the barriers, the Department of Work and Pensions (DWP) reviewed the Personal Capability Assessment (PCA) to transform it from a tool for determining entitlement to incapacity benefits to a more inclusive assessment of capability and of health-related interventions. The new PCA assesses what an individual can do and what interventions would help to break down the barriers that prevent them from working. By considering an individual's ability over a period of time rather than as a 'snapshot', it addressed the potential impact of conditions that fluctuate over time.

From 2008, and for new claimants only, a new Employment and Support Allowance (ESA) will replace Incapacity Benefit (IB) and Income Support paid on the grounds of incapacity. This will be structured to support and encourage people to access employment opportunities and will centre around drawing up a personal action plan focused on rehabilitation and work-related activity.

WHAT WORKS – THE EVIDENCE

It has been widely documented that work enhances the mental health and quality of life of people who experience mental health problems.[18,19] Work also provides benefits beyond that of an income, such as a means of structuring and occupying time, social identity and inclusion, a sense of purpose and personal achievement[20] and can result in a reduction in symptoms, increased leisure activities and self-esteem, and reduced dependency and relapse.[21,22] In many cases, appropriate support in getting back to work and a job can itself be a vital progression in recovery, helping people towards improved health and well-being as well as giving them greater control over their own health.[23] Repeated postponement in starting the process of returning to work can be a central factor in determining a unsuccessful outcome.

The research literature shows that models and approaches are more important than client characteristics in determining whether people with mental problems are able to work.[24] However, it is important that there is a range of vocational opportunities to meet the needs of all individuals, including those most disabled by their mental health problems. Services need to allow people to attain a range of personal goals, from full-time employment or education to volunteering to pre-vocational training, that support people towards increased independence and social inclusion, and also towards their individual aspirations.

DH[25] vocational commissioning guidance provides five key elements to a comprehensive range of vocational services for people with severe mental health problems:

1 clinical employment leads within secondary services who offer a clinical perspective on vocational rehabilitation
2 employment specialists integrated with clinical teams who identify vocational needs and support people into employment, education or voluntary work
3 public services as exemplar employers who can offer a wide range of employment opportunities
4 supported work opportunities that may be in open employment, social enterprises or a social firm where support is offered for as long as is required
5 local partnership arrangements between specialist and mainstream providers with appropriate commissioner input.

Early intervention services are important, as returning to a work pattern can be increasingly difficult when someone is unemployed and has a mental health problem. Rinaldi *et al.*[26] found that implementing supported employment within an early intervention service increases employment and education opportunities for patients within the service.

Research indicates that segregated sheltered workshops may help to increase people's confidence and skills and perhaps enable them to move on to some form of work, but they are relatively poor at enabling people to return to open employment. One of the risks attached to these workshops is that they often confirm a person's belief that they would not be able to manage in open employment and move-on rates have been poor.[27]

Findings showed that a sustained period of pre-vocational training before returning to work has limited outcomes beyond occupying the time of service users and does not enable people to access work. The Cochrane Review[28] found no evidence to suggest that those attending pre-vocational training were any more successful in securing open employment than were those receiving standard community or hospital care. However, services and professionals need to consider that offering structure and occupation to a person's day may be the appropriate goal for some people at specific points in their rehabilitation and may be their preference to standard hospital care.

In contrast, the Cochrane Review, which looked at 18 randomised controlled trials (RCTs), illustrated that there is strong evidence in favour of supported employment; more specifically, evidence-based supported employment (formerly known as the individual placement and support (IPS) approach) developed by Drake and Becker was recommended over other approaches such as sheltered workshops and pre-vocational training.

The IPS approach involves assessing vocational skills and preferences relatively quickly and then attempting to place people in employment settings that are consistent with their abilities and interests, where they can develop their skills in the work environment while being provided with ongoing support. Support is also provided to the employer and directly to the workplace if necessary in order to ensure maintenance of the placement. Research into the effectiveness of this approach shows that there are six operational principles, detailed by Bond,[29] which are:

➤ services should focus on paid employment with a primary goal of paid employment in integrated settings
➤ programmes should involve rapid job search and minimal pre-vocational training
➤ support should come from vocational workers based in clinical teams, with employment being an integral part of the overall care plan
➤ job searches should be driven by client preferences and choice
➤ there should be continual assessment of people's needs, with support adjusted as necessary and assistance in career progression
➤ access should be available to time-unlimited support once in work, which should be tailored to the person's individual needs.

As well as benefits, counselling could also be provided to help people maximise their welfare benefits.

The accuracy with which IPS is implemented can be measured using the Supported Employment Fidelity Scale. However, this is often not used by providers,[30] despite the consistency and outcome measure that it can offer. SESAMI[31] also found that the quality of the support provided is as important as its organisational features. The report suggests that combining IPS with motivation and confidence-building psychological input is critical, as is liaising with occupational health professionals so that screening procedures do not present difficulties.

With the advent of Foundation Trusts and the drive towards economic stability and evidence-based approaches, the IPS is an attractive option for services and local communities. Research has shown that there is a positive cost-benefit analysis for the individual over other alternative interventions.[32] While the costs to the taxpayer may exceed the economic benefits in the short term, there may be overall gains in the longer term. Similarly, supported employment is socially inclusive, which is a societal benefit that derives from employment interventions but not from most alternatives.[33]

MENTAL HEALTH AND HOUSING

There is a growing concern that the lack of appropriate housing is a major cause of delayed discharge from mental health inpatient care, while a lack of stable housing, or unsuitable housing, can lead to worsening mental health.[34] The SEU[35] found that people with mental health problems, compared with the general population, are one-and-a-half times more likely to live in rented accommodation, and alone, and are four times more likely to say that their health has been made worse by their housing circumstances. People are also twice as likely to say that they are dissatisfied with their accommodation or that its state of repair is poor.

Rent arrears and choice-based lettings: the challenges

Research commissioned by the Office of the Deputy Prime Minister (now the Department for Communities and Local Government, DCLG) found that possession action by social landlords more than doubled in the decade to 2003. By 2002–03, these were resulting in the eviction of around 26 000 tenants annually.[36] The vast majority of such repossessions are triggered by rent arrears. People with mental health problems are particularly vulnerable to accumulated arrears, may find it difficult to keep on top of their rent and housing benefit claims and are often unaware of the advice that is available. Indeed, one in four tenants with mental health problems has serious rent arrears and risks losing their home.[37] Eviction can mean that people are no longer eligible to access social housing and this can have a devastating impact on the individual and their carers. Effective mental health services can have a significant role in providing support and information during these stressful times.

A proactive, preventative approach with regular communication can also provide considerable benefits to housing providers. People may isolate themselves if feeling unwell, and this can frequently be a common trigger for rent arrears. Written correspondence can break down, so retaining verbal communication with the person is key – firstly to offer support, but also to ensure that the person understands what is going on with their rent account, and most importantly the steps taken to begin addressing it.

Along with the briefing on rent arrears management, Care Services Improvement Partnership (CSIP)[38] also published information on choice-based lettings (CBL) for people with mental health problems.[39] CBL schemes are being actively promoted by the Government and allow people to apply for available social housing accommodation, which is openly advertised. People can see the range of available properties and apply for any home to which they are matched – the successful bidder is the one with the highest priority under the scheme. However, people with mental health problems may face a number of difficulties in accessing the local CBL scheme because they are often unaware that the scheme is in operation and may find it difficult to navigate the system or bid for properties, particularly where the CBL systems are heavily based on information technology. People may also require additional advice and support to exercise choice and adopt a realistic home-hunting strategy.

People may initially seek advice and information about CBL from Social Services or even Health Services. It is helpful for health and social care staff to have a basic understanding of CBL as a system. Knowledge of local authority advice, support and information services, which a person can be signposted to, as well as who would be the first point of contact for someone wishing to access the local CBL scheme, is also key.

THE ROLE OF MENTAL HEALTH SERVICES

Mental health services have a crucial role to play in enabling people with severe mental health problems to gain and retain employment and improve community engagement. People with severe mental health problems can and do want to work but over half who are in contact with mental health services do not receive any help to find work, although they would like to receive it. In addition, it is clear that the expectations of health professionals play a key part in the aspirations of individuals.

COMMISSIONING SERVICES

Commissioners of mental health services need to work closely with these services and to ensure that they are following evidence-based approaches and policy guidelines. The DH[40-2] published three guidance documents for commissioners on vocational services, day-service modernisation and direct payments, and each details approaches to improve the reintegration of people with mental health problems into society. The Direct Payments guidance illustrates how people with mental health problems can be given control over their own lives by providing an alternative to social care services of a local council. The guidance on day services and vocational services complement this by refocusing efforts on providing opportunities for people with mental health problems to access more community services as well as to gain employment.

The underpinning commissioning principles for vocational services for people with severe mental health problems[43] are:

➤ priority is accorded to enabling people to retain and gain paid employment and mainstream education, including the provision of support to retain and gain employment/education
➤ where it is not possible, or there is an individual preference not to access paid employment, then mainstream educational opportunities or mainstream voluntary work is needed
➤ where the extent of support or supervision needs is high, then access to supported work opportunities is needed.

The needs of people from black and minority ethnic (BME) groups are invariably not adequately addressed by IPS services and women appear to be under-represented.[44] Commissioners should ensure equality of access and need to address the imbalances of provision while negotiating vocational outcomes and targets with services.

PARTNERSHIP WORKING

The principle of partnership working and integration into local communities is at the heart of achieving Foundation Trust status and also the social inclusion agenda. Vocational services and employment should be central when services are developing their philosophies of care and models of practice.

Any service modernisation and improvements in the opportunities for people with mental health problems needs to have close partnership working directed through strong leadership. Key local agencies to enable people with severe mental health problems to gain and retain paid employment, education, voluntary work and housing include Primary Care Trusts, Mental

Health Trusts, local authorities, Jobcentre Plus, Connexions, Learning and Skills Councils, Next Step, colleges, mainstream training organisations, volunteer bureaus, the voluntary sector and local housing associations.[45]

Partnership working between housing and mental health services is also paramount in reducing the difficulties caused by rent arrears and poor housing, as well as gaining information and access to choice-based lettings. The CSIP briefing[46] outlines the principles of effective joint working:

➤ referral and information-sharing protocols between agencies
➤ joint training to understand the pressure and challenges experienced by each other
➤ care co-ordination and communication with (potential) housing representation in Care Programme Approach (CPA) meetings
➤ Mental Health Trusts and Housing taking joint responsibility for ensuring that tenants have clear and comprehensive information about local support services
➤ joint reviews of service provision and agency practice
➤ involvement of services/vulnerable tenants in developing local housing strategies.

LEADERSHIP AND THE WORKFORCE

The importance of the provision of clear leadership originates from several sources. Local agencies may have specific roles in relation to enabling people with severe mental health problems to gain and retain paid employment, education or voluntary work. However, without clear local leadership and co-ordination, those agencies tend not to maximise knowledge, expertise and resources, which can lead to duplication of services and a lack of equity across areas.

Leadership within mental health services needs to provide a clear vision and direction to its workforce and ensure that they facilitate and enable the delivery of best practice and do not allow complacency or support outdated models of practice. As well as government policy initiatives, there are capabilities for practice that can be used for delivering modern services. The *Ten Essential Shared Capabilities*[47] offers a framework for all practitioners to achieve best practice and provides the building blocks for all staff in mental health services, whether professionally qualified or not.

An SEU report[48] found that the low expectations of health professionals can be a restriction to people accessing work. Unintentionally, professionals with such attitudes can reinforce the belief that people with a mental health problem should avoid trying to go back to paid work until they are fully recovered or without any symptoms of their diagnosis. This assumption fails to recognise the negative relationship between unemployment and poor mental health.[49] For many people, inactivity and lack of purpose compounds health problems and leads to longer-term absence from a job and an increased challenge in finding work.

Using the framework of the capabilities can provide a way of addressing some of these misunderstandings and attitudes. The importance of developing these skills and approaches in the mental health workforce is reflected through the initiatives of key professional bodies. For example, the Chief Nursing Officer's review of mental health nursing[50] has a central theme of social inclusion and recovery, as has the mental health strategy of the College of Occupational Therapists (COT).[51] It is vital that managers within services use the available evidence and messages when leading service delivery and staff training and that the principles are inherent in all aspects of care. Training on supported employment should be made available to staff and should focus on the quality of the employment support from a service user perspective as well as on organisational features. Ensuring that staff have appropriate training to deliver psychological preparation for work is also central to improving motivation and confidence, alongside job preparation and job search.[52]

CARE PROGRAMME APPROACH

The Care Programme Approach (CPA) is designed to assess and plan for the needs of people using specialist mental health services and should include everyone who is involved in the care of the individual. Mental health services should aim for the provision of vocational and social support to be embedded in the CPA, with full involvement of the service user,[53] and all mental health staff have a role in achieving this.

However, services do not routinely collect data on employment and there is limited evidence of occupational care planning within CPA. Despite there being high rates of unemployment for people with mental health problems, there are very low rates for service users being referred for vocational interventions – especially when these users are from a BME group.[54] Care co-ordinators, who have an overview of all aspects of the person's care and co-ordinate this, need to work beyond health services and include all areas in which the individual requires support, including vocational, social and housing support, and data collection needs to be a central aspect of the work. From a vocational perspective, this would include:

➤ establishing employment status on admission to hospital
➤ supporting job retention

➤ promoting involvement of carers and families
➤ identifying a lead contact on vocational and social issues in secondary care teams
➤ strengthening links to key local partners, in particular Jobcentre Plus and education providers
➤ promoting access to advice and support on benefits issues
➤ monitoring vocational outcomes for people on CPA
➤ monitoring the employment rates of people with mental health problems within their own organisation.

Covering these aspects of data and intervention within the CPA and the role of mental health staff will lead to improved vocational – and more broadly, social inclusion – outcomes.

CONCLUSION

There is an increasing evidence base for what works from individual, service and economic perspectives, and commissioners should respond positively to relevant information and guidance. Effective management and leadership are at the heart of delivering what users say they need, which in turn fulfils ambitions for the national policy agenda. Health professionals need broad training to address the psychological aspects of job preparation as well as the practical job preparation and job search activities that are part of supported employment, education and voluntary work. Staff should be supported in working beyond the boundaries of healthcare, looking to local partnerships and community engagement that enable the implementation of whole systems interventions that support people to gain control, hope and choice in their lives.

The association between meaningful activity, including work, and better health outcomes for people with mental health problems is proven. However, this is dependent on other factors, which are often interrelated. These would include, by necessity, decent housing and economic stability, such as access to relevant income and benefits. The Government, society, the individual, their families and friends all benefit from improved mental health outcomes. The final part of the jigsaw is the help and support available to enable people to move forward and mental health providers have a critical role in developing, delivering and implementing services that increase opportunities and aspirations.

REFERENCES

1 Bartley M. Unemployment and ill health: understanding the relationships. *J Epidemiol Community Health.* 1994; **48**: 333–7.

2 Warner R. *Recovery from Schizophrenia: psychiatry and political economy.* 2nd ed. Oxford: Oxford University Press; 1994.

3 Lewis G, Sloggett A. Suicide, deprivation and unemployment: record linkage study, *BMJ.* 1998; **317**: 1283–6.

4 Department of Health. *Safety First: five-year report of the national inquiry into suicide and homicide by people with mental illness.* London: Department of Health; 2001.

5 McLean C, Francis S. *Worklessness and Health: what do we know about the causal relationship?* London: Health Development Agency; 2004.

6 Waddell G, Burton A. *Is Work Good for Your Health and Wellbeing?* London: HMSO; 2006.

7 Bennett DH. Social forms of psychiatric treatment. In: Wing JK, editor. *Schizophrenia: towards a new synthesis.* London: Academic Press; 1978.

8 Office for National Statistics. *Labour Force Survey: estimated figures for adults aged 16–64, living in England.* London: Office for National Statistics; Spring 2005.

9 Social Exclusion Unit. *Mental Health and Social Exclusion.* London: Office of the Deputy Prime Minister; 2004.

10 Secker J, Grove B, Seebohm P. Challenging barriers to employment, training and education for mental health service users. *Journal of Mental Health.* 2001; **10**: 395–404.

11 South Essex Service User Research Group (SE-SURG), Secker J, Gelling L. Still dreaming: service users' employment, education and training goals. *J Ment Health.* 2006; **15**(1): 103–11.

12 Social Exclusion Unit. Op. cit.

13 Department of Work and Pensions. *A New Deal for Welfare: empowering people to work Green Paper.* London: Department of Work and Pensions; 2006.

14 Department of Health. *Our Health, Our Care, Our Say: a new direction for community services.* London: Department of Health; 2006.

15 Cabinet Office. *Reaching Out: an action plan on social exclusion.* London: Cabinet Office; 2006.

16 Department of Health/Department of Work and Pensions. *Vocational Services for People with Severe Mental Health Problems: commissioning guidance.* London: Department of Health; 2006.

17 Social Exclusion Unit. Op. cit.

18 Department of Health/Department of Work and Pensions. Op. cit.

19 Perkins R, Rinaldi M. Unemployment rates among people with long-term mental health problems. A decade of rising unemployment. *Psychiatr Bull.* 2002; **26**: 295–8.

20 Boardman J, Grove B, Perkins R, *et al.* Work and employment for people with psychiatric disabilities. *Br J Psychiatry.* 2006; **182**: 467–8.

21 Cook A, Razzano L. Vocational rehabilitation for persons with schizophrenia: recent research and implications for practice. *Schizophr Bull.* 2000; **26**: 87–103.

22 Bond GR, Resnik SG, Drake RE, *et al.* Does competitive employment improve non-vocational outcomes for people with severe mental illness? *J Consult Clin Psychol.* 2001; **69**(3): 489–501.

23 Department of Health. *Choosing Health: making healthy choices easier*. London: Department of Health; 2004.

24 Crowther RE, Marshall M, Bond GR *et al*. Helping people with severe mental illness to obtain work: systematic review. *BMJ*. 2001; **322**: 204–8.

25 Department of Health/Department of Work and Pensions. Op. cit.

26 Rinaldi M, Mcneil K, Firn M, *et al*. What are the benefits of evidence based supported employment for patients with first episode psychosis? *Psychiatr Bull*. 2004; **28**: 281–4.

27 Grove B. Mental health and employment. Shaping a new agenda. *J Ment Health*. 1999; **8**: 131–40.

28 Crowther R, Marshall M, Bond G, *et al*. *Vocational Rehabilitation for People with Severe Mental Illness* (Cochrane Review). In: The Cochrane Library, Issue 3, 2006 (Reprint from 2003).

29 Bond GR. Supported employment: evidence for an evidence-based practice. *Psychiatr Rehabil J*. 2004; **27**: 345–59.

30 SESAMI. *Social Inclusion through Employment Support for Adults with Mental Illness*. European Community Social Fund; 2006.

31 Ibid.

32 Cimera RE. The cost-efficiency of supported employment programs: a literature review. *J Vocat Rehabil*. 2000; **14**: 51–61.

33 Schneider J. Is supported employment cost effective? A review. *Int J Psychosoc Rehabil*. 2003; **7**: 145–56.

34 Care Service Improvement Partnership. *Improving the Effectiveness of Rent Arrears Management for People with Mental Health Problems*. London: National Social Inclusion Programme; 2006.

35 Social Exclusion Unit. Op. cit.

36 Office of the Deputy Prime Minister. *Improving the Effectiveness of Rent Arrears Management: good practice guidance*. London: Office of the Deputy Prime Minister; 2002.

37 Ibid.

38 Care Service Improvement Partnership. Op. cit.

39 Care Service Improvement Partnership. *Choice Based Lettings for People with Mental Health Problems*. London: National Social Inclusion Programme; 2006.

40 Department of Health 2001. Op. cit.

41 Department of Health. *From Segregation to Inclusion: commissioning guidance on day service for people with mental health problems*. London: Department of Health; 2006.

42 Department of Health. *Direct Payment for People with Mental Health Problems: a guide to action*. London: London: Department of Health; 2006.

43 Ibid.

44 SESAMI. Op. cit.

45 Department of Health/Department of Work and Pensions. Op. cit.

46 Care Service Improvement Partnership. *National Social Inclusion Programme 2nd Annual Report*. London: National Social Inclusion Programme; 2006.

47 Department of Health. *The Ten Essential Shared Capabilities: a framework for the whole of the mental health workforce*. London: London: Department of Health; 2005.

48 Social Exclusion Unit. Op. cit.

49 Perkins R, Rinaldi M. Op. cit.

50 Department of Health. *From Values to Action: the Chief Nursing Officer's review of mental health nursing.* London: London: Department of Health; 2006.

51 College of Occupational Therapists. *Recovering Ordinary Lives: the strategy for occupational therapy in mental health services for 2007–2017. A vision for the next ten years.* London: COT; 2006.

52 SESAMI. Op. cit.

53 Social Exclusion Unit. Op. cit.

54 Bertram M, Howard L. Employment status and occupational care planning for people using mental health services. *Psychiatr Bull.* 2006; **30**: 48–51.

CHAPTER 11

Devolving mental health social care: policy outcomes in Sweden and England

WENDY MAYCRAFT KALL

INTRODUCTION

'Do you trust mental health services?'[1] asked a Swedish newspaper in January 1997 when another scandal erupted concerning community-based living. Such headlines could just as easily have come from English newspapers where community mental healthcare scandals are also sadly familiar. Both Sweden and England developed similar policies to devolve mental health social care in the 1990s, with visions of different public-sector organisations working in harmony to co-ordinate client-centred services. Yet in both countries outcomes reported in the media have been policy confusion and declarations of failure. So can it be assumed that community-based social care resulted in the same 'failures' in both countries, or did the problems encountered have differing causes? This chapter will give an overview of the implementation of devolution policies in Sweden and England, and compare outcomes, focusing upon political steering and interactions between different levels of government.

REVISITING COMMUNITY CARE: DEVOLVING SOCIAL CARE

The policies of devolving social care had similar origins in both countries. De-hospitalisation and increased community care had been debated since the 1950s, although the focus remained medical. By the 1980s, both countries faced the dual issues of public-sector financial crises, coupled with public debate and political rhetoric concerning normalised living and community care. The devolution of mental health social care was perceived as a solution to these issues.

Devolving mental healthcare involved separating medical and social care functions. Medical care would remain under health authority control while social care would transfer to local authority social services departments. In Sweden, community-based social care was introduced by the Government Proposition (Bill) 1993–94: 218, The Conditions of the Mentally Disordered (Psykiskt stördas villkor), implemented on 1 January 1995. In England, devolution resulted from the National Health Service (NHS) and Community Care Act (1990), enacted 1 April 1993. The broad aims of devolution were the same in both countries:

➤ local authorities assumed financial and service responsibility for mental health social care and support
➤ the mentally ill and disabled would live normal lives in the community
➤ asylum closure and community care would reduce expenditure.[2]

EVALUATING POLICY OUTCOMES

Over a decade has passed since community-based social care was introduced. There has been significant media coverage and political rhetoric of 'failures' and scandals in both countries. Mental health social care is a complex subject sitting on the boundaries between different territorial (central/local) and sectoral (health/social care) priorities and objectives. But have the outcomes been the same? Petersson contends that the political management of policy implementation can be evaluated by four mechanisms of political influence and control:

➤ rules and regulation
➤ finance
➤ organisation
➤ staffing.[3]

RULES AND REGULATIONS: FORMAL STEERING MECHANISMS

The main instruments of government influence are legislation and other regulations governing activities. Devolution of mental health aimed to split social care, which transferred to local authorities from medical care, which remained a health authority responsibility.

Sweden

In Sweden, medical and psychiatric care is governed by the Health and Medical Care Act 1982 (*Hälsö och sjukvårdslagen 1982: 763*). Social care is regulated by the Social Services Act 2001 (*Socialtjänstlagen 2001: 453*) and the Disability Services and Support Act 1993 (*Lagen om stöd och service till vissa funktionshindrade 1993: 387*). The mental health reform assumed that most clients would receive statutory services under the Disability Services and Support Act. However, this disability perspective was not evident in practice; a follow-up study concluded that 74% of clients received no Disability Act services; instead the weaker Social Services Act was employed (84%).[4]

The Social Services Act is framework legislation whereby broad aims are specified and local authorities decide what/how services are delivered. The Act requires local authorities to:

➤ provide decent living standards
➤ inventory individual needs including outreach work to identify need
➤ plan services and co-ordinate with other agencies.[5]

The Board of Health and Welfare's report revealed that only 50% of local authorities have adequate planning information and most lack steering, planning and quality control systems. Responsibilities are poorly defined with negligible user input. One-third of social care services lack defined objectives, almost two-thirds lack adequate service plans and three-quarters have no quality control systems.

TABLE 11.1 Adequacy of local authority planning and monitoring systems[6]

Local authority has adequate systems for	Yes %	No %
Objective setting	61	39
Service planning	39	61
Quality control	23	77

The lack of specific rules and targets resulted in confusion within the local authorities. Many social workers did not compile individual needs-based plans, instead merely informing clients of existing services on a 'take it or leave it' basis.

England

In England, medical/psychiatric care is regulated by the Mental Health Act 1983. De-hospitalisation was not a new idea, but in the past local authorities had few incentives to finance community-based social care owing to the 'perverse incentive' whereby residential care was financed by central government.

Devolution of social care occurred via the National Health Service (NHS) and Community Care Act 1990, establishing principles of community-based mental health social care. Following scandals and criticisms, New Labour's Health Secretary, Frank Dobson, declared in 1998 that community care had 'failed' and would be dismantled.[7] Yet although the emphasis changed, there was no fundamental policy U-turn. Community care was re-labelled as social care and a plethora of new initiatives followed relating to mental health social care (too many to discuss all in detail here). White Papers such as *Modernising Mental Health* and *Modernising Social Services* made mental health a stated priority, although the new Mental Health Act was delayed. The discourse changed to emphasise social exclusion, employment, quality, cost-effectiveness, risk management, coercion and greater central control. Government policy placed an onus on social care services to meet a wide variety of sometimes conflicting needs and expectations of service users, communities, taxpayers, central government, health authorities and external regulators while delivering low-cost, high-quality 'safe, sound and supportive' services that meet government's targets.[8]

The New Labour Government substantially increased regulation, inspection and control. The Care Standards Act 2000 brought social care professionals under central control. The Health and Social Care Act 2003 created the Commission for Social Care Inspection as well as introducing league tables, targets and star-ratings for social care. Therefore the UK Government used top-down steering and control strategies to produce greater standardisation and control, with programmes evaluated in terms of measurable outputs.

FINANCE: WHO CONTROLS SOCIAL CARE RESOURCES?

Devolution of mental health social care required resources and involved major new financial commitments for local authorities in an area not always prioritised by local politicians.

Sweden

In Sweden, most local authorities' finance comes from local income taxes and these vary according to each authority's expenditure, as Sweden does not have national income tax rates. Local authority income comprises 69.5% local taxes and 14.1% government grants; the remainder is made up of fees, charges, rents and other income.[9] Higher expenditure is directly visible to local taxpayers and politicians. Therefore balancing expectations of taxpayers, users, partners and other actors is complex and can create conflict.

In order to ease the transition and develop joined-up services, central government provided pump-priming financing for three years. However, devolution coincided with a recession, high unemployment and reduced public-sector finance. A review carried out by The National Mental Health Co-ordinator (*Psykiatrisamordnare*)[10] asserts that some health authorities regarded devolution of social care as an opportunity to reduce psychiatry services and budgets. Financial constraints meant that the vision of joined-up services was difficult to realise. The short-term government financing led to many services starting as temporary projects involving external partners – including primary care, Social Insurance (*Försäkringskassan*) and Employment (*Arbetsförmedlingen*) agencies – assuming that shared financial responsibility would continue. Yet when government financing ended, most non-local authority partners withdrew, leaving local authorities with sole financial responsibility.[11] Therefore, although government finance enabled the initial development of creative and flexible services, there were negative consequences; mental health failed to become a budgetary priority among local politicians, and the other partners' roles were unclear.

England

In England, local authority finance is more directly controlled by the government: only 25% of revenue expenditure is financed by locally determined taxes; 54% comes from government grants and 21% from business rates, fixed by central government.[12] Therefore central government directly determines the levels of finance available for local authority services. Devolving mental health social care led to many costs transferring to local authorities without adequate compensation. Langan asserts that community care evolved as a client-dumping mechanism; other services redefined their 'core business' and reduced budgets by transferring clients to the vaguely defined concept of the 'community' whereas the reality was Social Services departments struggling to cope.[13]

Considerable cost pressures remain. Service commissioners must balance conflicting interests to deliver services that meet user and community needs, promote independence, provide choice within the context of local care markets, and provide high-quality yet cost-effective services. Commissioners must balance increased costs from rising demand, rising salary costs, and increased quality expectations. Additionally the National Health Service (NHS) financial crisis creates boundary disputes as NHS bodies seek to withdraw from joint funding arrangements. Many local authorities restrict eligibility as a gatekeeping method to reduce costs.[14] The 'Old Maid'[15] game is played as organisations attempt to avoid being left with responsibility for costly mental health clients.

Organisation: creating joined-up service structures

The organisational structures created for the delivery of mental health social care services are an important aspect in evaluating the outcomes of social care reforms and the respective roles and priorities of central and local governments.

Sweden

Sweden has a tradition of relatively independent local government, with central government often being reluctant to steer local authorities. Legislation usually contains general policy aims for local authorities to interpret and implement. Many Swedish local authorities provide mental health services directly to clients, although the use of private companies is increasing. However, there were great variations in local authorities' perception of their task. Some local authorities created specialist mental health units while others interpreted 'integration' and 'normalisation' to mean the assimilation of social care within existing structures, resulting in fragmented and blurred lines of responsibility. In 53% of local authorities, responsibility was divided between several departments, e.g. Individual and Family Services; Disability Services; Elderly Care, etc.[16] The government's pump-priming finance also caused internal organisational problems as the temporary projects limited long-term, strategic decision-making. When government finance ran out, specialist teams were often dismantled, and expertise was lost.[17] Services lacked long-term planning horizons and were not incorporated into political priorities and mainstream social services, organisational and decision-making structures.

Internal co-ordination continues to be poor as services are often not politically prioritised at local levels. Services frequently lack mental health specialists and some small local authorities have no mental health-trained staff. Complex, fragmented organisations have reduced service accessibility. Additionally, information concerning mental health clients is not always disseminated within the social services' organisation.[18]

In Sweden, external co-ordination has proved difficult. Each local authority determines its own levels of formal co-operation with other agencies, most commonly with health authority psychiatric services. Despite powers to form joint organisations, few have been created. Formal co-operation with central government agencies such as Social Insurance (*Försäkringskassen*) and Employment (*Arbetsförmedlingen*) agencies has been poor. The Board of Health and Welfare concluded that only 27% of local authorities had adequate joint planning arrangements with other agencies, with many being unclear about how to co-ordinate services. The Board advised the Government to provide more guidance about service co-ordination, in particular to define/resolve boundary disputes between health and local authorities.[19] Organisationally, Swedish governments have provided only loose steering and control over social care. Services have developed locally, in a bottom-up manner, with little direction from central government. Many local authorities were uncertain of their role and lacked the necessary skills to create suitable organisations.

England

Since New Labour came to power, organisational complexity and flexibility has increased in England, with a plethora of new organisational groupings created. Mental health services may be integrated with other social care functions or separate departments may exist for mental health clients. Services can be located within local authorities, health authorities or in multi-disciplinary care trusts. However, local authorities are not always direct care providers. Services are organised via the 'mixed economy of care', whereby local authorities commission care from external providers such as private care companies, independent specialist organisations or the voluntary sector. Increasingly, joint mental health and social care trusts have been formed to co-ordinate partnerships between NHS, local authorities, private sector and voluntary services. There are 74 Mental Health Trusts and currently 10 Primary Care Trusts.[20]

The Government envisaged partnership working and joined-up organisations for social care. While many formal partnerships with the NHS have been formed, establishing partnership working has been complex and the majority of partnerships are described as a 'challenge'. Complex delivery systems created initial gaps, duplication and conflicts between clinical and social care values.[21] A survey by Huxley *et al.* of over 300 mental health social workers found that co-ordination with the NHS was complex, resulting in confused organisations. Compatibility between NHS and local authorities was poor, with different priorities, information technology systems, procedures and training. Poor integration increased the administrative burden. In some cases, social workers maintained *both* paper and computer records to comply with both systems.[22] Social services departments became forced into reactive roles, taking on new tasks dictated by central government and health authorities. Services were redefined to accommodate health priorities while social services lost direct provision roles to the independent sector. Therefore, organisations became vulnerable to shifting priorities and financial constraints of other partners.

STAFF: RECRUITING PROFESSIONALS AND COMPETENCE FOR MENTAL HEALTH

Experienced, qualified staff are essential to social care. For mental health, this required a new social care culture to replace previous medical care models.

Sweden

The introduction of community-based social care envisages access to knowledgeable staff, yet local authorities received little personnel guidance. Initially recruitment was difficult, as mental health services were considered uncertain and unattractive. Many local authorities solved recruitment problems by using supernumerary staff who had not volunteered for social care, and transfers of former health authority staff, experienced in medical rather than social care. The majority of social care staff had few formal qualifications and many services lacked a specific *social* focus. Social care had low status, with little direct involvement from professional groups and, in particular, the role of qualified social workers was undefined:

➤ no social work role in the legislation was created – individual local authorities determined the social work role, leading to wide variations
➤ organisational fragmentation led to social work's not being responsible for internal/external co-ordination between units/organisations. Politicians and senior managers did not generally expect social workers to be responsible for strategic oversight, individual planning, and co-ordination
➤ staff roles were not defined, especially the division of responsibilities between social workers and care assistants
➤ mental health work was unattractive to social workers and few volunteered for mental health services.[23]

TABLE 11.2 Social care assessment – do services meet client needs?[24]

Client need	Needs met %	Needs unmet %	Don't know %
Housing	66	16	18
Daily activity services	36	26	38
Physical and mental health	34	19	47
Dental health	27	3	70

In Sweden, social workers do not occupy a central role for strategic oversight and co-ordination. A random survey of 462 individual cases by the Board of Health and Welfare revealed that social workers were frequently unaware of services being provided by other sections within social services and whether identified needs were being met. Surprisingly in only 34% of cases were clients' physical and mental health needs known to be met, and huge gaps were revealed in social services' knowledge of the effectiveness of services provided.

It was surprising that a major social policy reform in Sweden does not appear to have created a specific role for the main social care profession, social work.

There are several explanations of why social work had a limited role:

➤ lack of mental health knowledge: 50% of social workers lack mental health training. Swedish social work degrees do not prepare staff for mental health work, especially relating to evidence-based methods. Social work is not a protected job title, the government does not control training, and there is no specialist mental health qualification. Social workers were not a prioritised group for training finance and the majority received no training.[25]

➤ bottom-up steering failed to create a distinct social work role: the Government's framework legislation did not specify qualifications for social care staff; the 'social' element of social care was never defined. Competence was often bought in using former health authority employees, paradoxically relying on staff trained in medical rather than social care. Local authorities' 'hands off' policies and the initial projects meant that mental health remained outside mainstream services and permanent local authority staff had little contact with mental health. This may have created reluctance among social workers to become involved beyond traditional authorisation roles.

➤ joined-up services v. cultural conflicts: the seamless, joined-up services envisaged by the Government failed to materialise; co-operation between local authorities, health authorities and other agencies was poor and professional conflicts arose. Markström's study found that unclear responsibilities resulted in professionally subordinate roles and lower status for social care staff. Despite asylum and inpatient bed closures, health authorities actually reduced outpatient care with 6% staff cuts.[26] Poor cross-boundary communication hampered professional co-operation between psychiatry and social services. Social Services departments have collective, committee-based decision-making cultures, with final decisions taken by politicians. Thus social workers lacked professional autonomy in negotiations with healthcare professions, despite being forced to accept responsibility for costs.[27] Therefore 'partnership' was often one-sided, with social care as the weaker partner.

England

In England, central government regulates and controls the social care workforce. The legal obligation to appoint specialist-approved social workers existed in the Mental Health Act 1983. The National Health Service and Community Care Act 1990 also created a mental health social work role, with local authority social workers responsible for planning and co-ordinating community services using the Care Programme Approach (CPA). However, poor communication and co-ordination in the community led to a number of mental health inquiries and, under New Labour, the emphasis changed from community reintegration to danger management. The new staff care role was based on risk management strategies and legal powers such as assertive outreach, risk assessment and community treatment orders. The Government has also emphasised staff roles in assessing/managing risk.[28] The changing nature and role of social care policy had a major impact on the social care workforce. The original vision of social workers supporting and caring was replaced with one where they held policing, monitoring and enforcement roles.

Recruitment of mental health social care staff in England remains problematic; 92% of local authorities experience recruitment difficulties and staff turnover is high.[29] Central control over staff has increased without additional professional recognition; many care assistants earn the minimum wage.[30] Services are co-ordinated by a care manager responsible for assessing individual user needs and developing care packages of public private and voluntary services to meet identified needs. Care managers must plan community mental health services and co-ordinate with health authorities. Although specific roles vary, the main tasks include:

➤ need assessment
➤ co-ordination with other partners
➤ consultation with users and carers
➤ negotiation and communication with service providers
➤ monitoring quality and costs.

In addition, there are general legal duties for approved social workers to provide statutory aftercare under the Mental Health Act 1983, supporting and monitoring mental health clients and arranging compulsory hospital readmission if necessary.[31]

In England, social care staff, especially social workers, have increasingly come under government control. The Care Standards Act 2001 created the General Social Care Council (GSCC) with the remit to regulate social care staff. Social work degrees must be approved by the GSCC, and social work has become a protected job title. All social workers must register and meet the

GSCC's requirements regarding qualifications, health, character and ethics. The GSCC can strike off social workers who fail to meet these standards.[32] The government's centralised control over social care staff can be seen as risk-reduction and blame-avoidance strategies. However, government control of social care also represents a deprofessionalisation of social work's autonomy in a manner that would be difficult to envisage applied to other professions such as medicine.

Mental health is envisaged as a joined-up service, with social care staff responsible for co-ordination between other services and sectors. Many social care staff are employed outside traditional local authority settings in multi-disciplinary agencies. Despite the formal legislative recognition of non-medical needs, joined-up working has proved difficult and cultural conflicts have arisen between medical and social care. Social care staff in joint organisations have became isolated, leading to high stress levels. It is perceived that medical cultures and models dominated services while social care has lower status and remains underdeveloped and underfunded. Multi-disciplinary organisations, such as Community Mental Health Services, although in theory joint services, tend to prioritise medical care.[33]

THE FUTURE: POLICY CONVERGENCE?

In November 2006, the Swedish Mental Health Co-ordinator reported on the state of mental health services, concluding that problems of social segregation persist. Most mental health clients exist on society's margins, dependent on benefits and with poor physical health. Clients lack access to co-ordinated, individualised, evidence-based social care services and many joined-up services lack co-ordination. However, the emphasis remains on care and support, with authorities urged to reduce measures that violate client integrity. Many local authorities must improve services and knowledge. The main recommendations relating to mental health social care were for:

➤ housing needs to be addressed with suitable services
➤ improved rehabilitation with access to study, work and activities
➤ high-quality, evidence-based care
➤ improved user and carer influence
➤ improved co-ordination and communication between partners
➤ enhanced national co-ordination, with central government improving steering and guidance as well as clarifying aims and eligibility under the Disability Act
➤ better co-ordination between local and health authorities, with boundary disputes being replaced by shared responsibility.[34]

In England, improving mental health social care is also problematic. In January 2007, the Commission for Social Care Inspection (CSCI) reported that, although services are modernising, the Government's stated ambitions remain unachieved. The main issues raised for future improvement mirror the findings of previous reports, including:

➤ financial problems, especially in joint services
➤ recruitment and retention problems
➤ underdevelopment of care markets
➤ lack of service information, choice and user influence
➤ increased pressure on individuals, carers and families.

The CSCI contends that the future of social care is uncertain, especially as responsibility for services appears to be shifting from the state to individuals.[35] In addition, the UK government relaunched its controversial Mental Health Bill in 2006, with new implications for social care. The risk management approach is evident, with an extension of forced community treatment, including restrictions to individual freedom – such as curfews, and requirements to reside at particular addresses, submit to medical examination or refrain from specified conduct.

Discussion: similar policies – similar outcomes?

We can see from the previous sections that, although policies may have been similar, the implementation and outcomes of mental health social care in Sweden and England differ. England has used centralised, top-down steering and control mechanisms over policy, finance and staffing, perhaps reflecting the greater central power and weaker powers of local authorities in England. There was a drive to create uniformity through standards and targets, yet accountability remains unclear, with policy/control functions separated from operational responsibilities. This often results in a circular blame game: local authorities blame failures on central targets and restrictions; whereas central government denies responsibility for 'operational issues'. In Sweden, ironically, pump-priming government finance created difficulty in mental health reform and services failed to become consolidated as mainstream local political priorities while they were run as temporary projects. The Government provided only framework legislation, allowing local authorities to formulate implementation strategies. However, this created wide variations in service ambition with finance dependent on local politicians' priorities. Mental health often became marginalised among the local government's competing interests, with politicians and senior managers lacking experience and knowledge of mental health.

Organisational fragmentation was a problem in both countries, and creating joined-up services between health and social care caused problems. Although joint working was an ambitious vision, in reality it was difficult to manage the interfaces between the different organisational cultures, structures, systems, financing priorities and professional interests. Despite devolution's aim of creating separate social expertise, medical culture tended to dominate organisations and social care became the junior partner. In England, service organisation was complex because of the pressure of the 'mixed economy' of social care markets where local authorities were responsible for services yet were not direct service producers. Even in Sweden, where many services were directly produced, decentralisation reforms with devolved management and budgeting functions created fragmentation and unclear service accountability, with no part of the organisation being designated with overall responsibility.

There were also staffing problems in both countries, with difficulties in recruiting social care staff. However, the political response varied. In England, top-down steering was again utilised, with centralised control over staff training and registration and a statutory role for social work, whereas in Sweden, there was no formal control over social care staffing and social workers in particular have no specified role. One conclusion would be that the mental health social care reforms were politically driven rather than profession driven. Professional conflicts emerged, with medical services dominant and social care forced into subordinate roles. The reforms aimed to recognise social rather than medical care needs, yet social aspects of care and the expertise required to deliver them were never defined.

When it comes to the future of social care services, England and Sweden face many similar problems, with issues of user influence, organisation, co-ordination, staffing and finance to be resolved. The scandals relating to mental health have increased political pressures in both countries to improve services and support in the community, but will identical methods be employed? Although the Swedish Mental Health Co-ordinator has recommended increased government guidance, it is doubtful whether this recommendation envisages the level of central control seen in England. At the moment, there is little evidence that Sweden will be adopting the English policing and surveillance methods in social care; locally determined services based on support and trust appear to be the Swedish strategies. The evidence of the past decade is that, despite similar aims, different implementation strategies for local authority mental health services will evolve in each country.

REFERENCES

1 Vidlund S. Läsarna rasar mot psykvården, *Aftonbladet*. 26 January 2007. Available at: http://deliverye.aftonbladet.se/vss/nyheter/story/0,2789,985629,00.html (accessed 2 February 2007) (author's translation).

2 *Regeringens proposition 1993–94*: 218. Psykist stördas villkor: 7–16. National Health Service and Community Care Act. London: HMSO; 1990: section III.

3 Petersson O. *Statsbyggnad: den offentliga maktens organisation* (5:e upplagen), Stockholm: SNS förlag; 2005: 31–46.

4 Statistics produced by the Swedish Board of Health and Welfare, the regulatory agency for health and social care. *Socialstyrelsen Kommunernas insatser för personer med psykiska funktionshinder: slutrapport från en national tillsyn 2002–2004*. Stockholm: Socialstyrelsen; 2005: 158.

5 See discussion in the Government Official Report (Statens Offentliga Utredning): SOU 2006: 100 *Ambition och Ansvar: Nationell strategi för utveckling av samhällets insatser till personer med psykiska sjukdomar och funktionshinder – slutbetänkande av nationell psykiatrisamordning*. Stockholm: Socialdepartement 2006; 104–5, 155–6.

6 *Socialstyrelsen*. Op. cit. pp. 59–81.

7 BBC. Care in the Community to be scrapped. BBC news online: 17 January 1998. Available at: http://news.bbc.co.uk/2/hi/uk_news/48168.stm (accessed 18 January 2007).

8 Department of Health. *Modernising Mental Health Services: safe, sound and supportive*. London: The Stationery Office; 1998.
Department of Health. *Modernising Social Services: promoting independence; improving protection; raising standards*. London: The Stationery Office; 1998.

9 Statistics from: *Sveriges Kommuner och Landsting*. The Economy Report: on Swedish Municipal and County Council Finances. Stockholm: 2005; 12.

10 In October 2003, the Swedish Government appointed a National Mental Health Co-ordinator to lead a three-year official commission of inquiry into mental health medical and social care. The Commission's task was to examine issues of organisation, coordination, resources, staffing and rehabilitation and to make preliminary reports as well as final recommendations (Kommittédirektiv 2003: 133. En Nationell Psykiatrisamordnare).

11 SOU 2006: 100. Op. cit. pp. 88–90.

12 Provisional out-turn for 2005–06. Department of Communities and Local Government. *Local Government Finance: key facts England 2006*. London: Department of Communities and Local Government; November 2006.

13 Langan M. Social services: managing the third way. In: Clarke J, Gerwirtz S, McLaughlin E, editors. *New Managerialism, New Welfare?* London: Sage; 2000: 156–7.

14 Commission for Social Care Inspection. *The State of Social Care in England 2005–2006*. London: Commission for Social Care Inspection; 2007: xi–xii, 59–60.

15 'Old Maid' is a traditional card game where players must avoid being left with the Old Maid card.

16 Markström U. *Den svenska psykiatrireformen: bland brukare, eldsjälar och byråkrater*. Umeå: Boréa: 2003: 183, 223; Socialstyrelsen 2005. Op. cit. p. 49.

17 Markström U. Op. cit. pp. 240–5; Interview with social worker, Mental Health Team, 27 March 2006.

18 SOU 2006: 100. Op. cit. pp. 157–66.

19 *Socialstyrelsen* 2005. Op. cit. pp. 84–92, 192–3.

20 Statistics from www.nhs.uk (accessed 31 January 2007).

21 Social Services Inspectorate. *Treated as People: an overview of mental health services from a social care perspective 2002–04*. London: Commission for Social Care Inspection; 2004. pp. 22–7.

22 Huxley P, Evans S, Gately C, *et al*. Stress and pressure in mental health social work: the worker speaks. *Br J Soc Work*. 2005; **35**(7): 1070–1.

23 *Socialstyrelsen* 2005. Op. cit. pp. 177–85; Markström U. Op. cit. pp. 184, 225.

24 Statistics: *Socialstyrelsen* 2005. Op. cit. p. 16.

25 Ibid. pp. 141–6.

26 Markström U. Op. cit. pp. 184–206, 260.

27 Sandelin G. Kunskap viktigt när socialtjänsten ska möta psykiatrin. SSR Tidning. *Socionomen*. 1996; **3**: 47.

28 Kemshall H. *Risk, Social Policy and Welfare*, Buckingham: Open University Press; 2002. pp. 90–102.

29 Huxley P, Evans S, Gately C, *et al*. Op. cit. pp. 1065–72.

30 See, for example: Batty D. Social care staff: the issue explained. *The Guardian*; 6 January 2004. Humphries P. Training investment blasted by underpaid social workers. *The Guardian*; 15 February 2002.

31 Available at: www.communitycare.co.uk (accessed 18 January 2007).

32 Information from the General Social Care Council. Available at: www.gscc.org.uk (accessed 18 January 2007).

33 See Social Services Inspectorate. Op. cit. pp. 28–30. MIND. *Social Care and Mental Health: MIND and current developments in adult social care*. MIND response to government Green Paper on social care. 2005; 3, 9. Available at: www.mind.org.uk/NR/rdonlyres/6A3CFEAE-3127-4235-B384643252245457/3154/socialcare.pdf (accessed 26 June 2006).

34 SOU 2006: 100. Op. cit. pp. 20–47.

35 Commission for Social Care Inspection. Op. cit. pp. x–xiii.

CHAPTER 12

Mental health in Europe: the Green Paper

JOHN BOWIS

'Wir haben in diesen letzten Wochen unsere Sprachlösigkeit überwunden und sind jetzt dabei, den aufrecten Gang zu erlernen.'

'In these last weeks, we have found our voice again and have learned once more to walk with our head held high.'

Stefan Heym – Alexanderplatz, East Berlin, November 1989.

Stefan Heym's November 1989 words to the vast crowd of East Berliners who had come together to oust a cruel regime should be our guide as we overturn and reform elements of mental health practice in Europe, which can so often be resource-inadequate and unthinkingly cruel. We need to bring mental health to standards of care, treatment, therapy, rehabilitation and patient involvement that we would expect of the best physical health systems. We can warmly welcome and endorse this Green Paper on Mental Health. We now look for swift and comprehensive proposals to translate the good words into effective legislative and codifying action.

The mental health challenge is to transform systems, attitudes and opportunities. For the past 40 years we have been emerging from a dark age of mental disorder practice. In some parts of our continent there has been the abuse of psychiatry; in others, an internment concept of asylum, which too often soothed the public's sensitivities with an 'out of sight, out of mind' institutionalisation, while doing little to help patients recover and rehabilitate; in others again, an overdependence on medication; in many, a reliance on prison rather than hospital; in none, a real understanding of mental health promotion.

We like to think we have moved on from the human rights abuses of mentally ill patients. And in many ways, we have. We still have debates about compulsory treatment; discharge or sectioning decisions are sometimes unsound; patient abuse is from time to time exposed in residential care; arguments abound on vexed and conflicting rights of patients, families and communities. But by and large, we have fewer locks and bolts, more patient choice and consent, legal checks and balances to see that the patient's civil rights are not abused.

Yet we still live in the dark age in at least one respect – stigma. It is rampant in all our countries and stigma is a human rights abuse, unintentional, born out of fear based on ignorance, but just as damaging to the individual as any other form of abuse. Living with mental illness is tough enough, without the added burden and pain of rejection and stigmatisation.

In calling for the Commission to develop its Green Paper into a Framework for Mental Health, we need to base such a policy on the facts about mental disorder and the Lisbon Agenda imperative for an increased recognition of the value of investment in mental well-being.

Underlying our policy are the facts:

➤ mental disorders are the fastest growing health burden, with unipolar depression the leading disorder

➤ 450 million people in our world live with a neurological or mental disorder

➤ one in four of us will be affected in our lifetime

➤ 121 million of us have depression – three in every 100 of us every year

➤ one million people in our world commit suicide and 10 million try to do so each year

➤ neuropsychiatric disorders are responsible for one-third of disabilities, 15% of inpatient costs, nearly one-quarter of drugs costs, half the caseload of social workers; and, in the United Kingdom alone, over 90 million days lost at work each year

➤ people are living longer and, on the whole, healthier lives, but in their later years a growing number of them become frail of body and mind

➤ carers – of a child, an adult or an elderly relative – have not been helped to adapt to the new community care of people with mental health problems

➤ drug addiction and crime, drunkenness, accidents, absenteeism, vandalism, disruptive pupils, rough sleepers, and many of society's 'problems' in fact link to mental health problems.

If we do not invest in the right range of services – inpatient, acute, long-stay, secure, medium-secure, day-care, domiciliary care and the trained staff for each – we shall not cure, care for or rehabilitate those who are ill now. If we do not invest in a mentally healthy life for our citizens, then the graph will continue rapidly to climb, in numbers and in cost. If we do not invest in bringing understanding about mental health and mental disorders, then budgets will remain pitiful and stigma and prejudice will be rampant.

Patients and service users are steadily and rightly moving centre-stage. They will be better informed, be more involved in decisions affecting them and will use their new rights to bypass sluggish services and effect change. They need to be seen as partners in their own treatment plans but also in service planning. Health professionals need to do what the best do in most areas of healthcare – explain and consult before decisions are taken. Then the patient will not just respect their professional judgement but would also, perhaps, understand a little more what was wrong and be a little less apprehensive about what was being done to them. That is right in human rights terms; it also makes for better compliance with and outcome from the treatment and care programme.

There has been a steady move from remote institution care to community services. This has applied to people with long-term and sometimes severe disorders and people with learning disability. To be successful, such services need adequate resources and multi-disciplinary teamwork. They also need to convince the public that such methods work for both patients and communities. Lurid media stories of patients being discharged and causing harm to themselves or others can undo years of work towards a more humane system and show how crucial proper checks and balances are. So can public uncertainty as to whether someone who may be behaving 'oddly' in the street is being adequately supervised.

There are five key flaws in our mental health system:
➤ the inadequacy of community services
➤ the failure to listen to service users and their carers
➤ the inability or unwillingness of different agencies to work together
➤ serious underfunding
➤ a policy for mental health promotion that is, in most countries, notable by its almost complete absence.

Someone with mental health problems needs a one-stop shop with one organisation ensuring contact, access to medical care, housing and other social care needs, income, legal services and rehabilitation. In other words, a single purchasing agency for all the person's needs and a trusted friend who knew his or her way around the provider organisations. That must go hand in hand with the skills and dedication of doctors, therapists and nurses, research scientists, managers of hospitals, clinics and community teams and the support of advocacy non-government organisations (NGOs). But, if one is ill or recovering from illness, one needs the security of a home, not in the isolation of high-rise flats on run-down estates, but in communities where the living environment will be part of the support and stability one needs. One needs access to activities that will aid recovery, support from family and neighbours. All these are just as important as medication or therapy sessions but organising that range of support may be beyond one, at least for the time being.

So many of us are going to need this enlightened care. Scientific and societal advances have brought new challenges and new costs in mental health and social care. A healthier, longer-living population means later years of high dependency, often with mental as well as physical frailty. Lifestyle, education and work pressures, changes in family structures, isolation, forced population movements, can all trigger mental health problems – psychoses, neuroses and often with an addiction link. New drugs, therapies and treatments have come at an escalating cost; new costs accompany new beds, centres, day care and community teams. And policy changes on where and when to treat and care have often added uncertainty to the standard problems of lack of understanding and inadequate resources, together leading to prejudice and the breeding grounds of stigma.

The crucial question is how to divert more political attention and then financial resources to mental health. Mental health really only penetrates the political and public mind when there is a crisis. In the UK, we achieved more progress on mental health, in terms of cash, initiatives and reforms, when one man jumped into the lion's den at London Zoo and another stabbed a stranger on the Underground, than at any other time, because colleagues across Government saw the need to do something and press, Parliament, public and NGOs clamoured for it. But it was at a price – the price of lowered public confidence and increased stigma.

Mental health promotion does not even benefit in that way from negative stories. There is little understanding by governments, politicians or even health service planners of mental health promotion. The main reason is that they have no idea what it is about or why they should be interested. Mental health suffers from a quadruple whammy. There is no constant public, professional and media pressure on government and health service managers to do more, spend more, achieve more. Unlike heart disease or AIDS or cancer, with mental illness there is little understanding of what can be done to treat, cure and rehabilitate. There is even less understanding of what can be done to prevent mental illness and promote mental health. And there are few outcome measurements that Health departments and managers – much less the public and politicians – can understand. Governments, employers, trade unions, schools, colleges, local councils and communities, families and individuals all need to be helped to understand the role they can play in ensuring mental well-being and so prevent, reduce or mitigate mental health problems.

Our challenge as policy-makers is to understand what it means to have a mental health problem. It almost certainly means that one is labelled, patronised, despised, feared and, to a greater or lesser extent, segregated – in society, within our family, at work, at play and even within our health and social services. In a perverse reversal, one can hide but one cannot run; one cannot perform; one cannot contribute to society as one would wish; one cannot lead full and fulfilling lives as one would want.

Then we have to accept our policy-making responsibilities. A service which does not gain professional, public and political support fails patients and their families doubly. It fails to treat and care adequately and it prompts a downward spiral of public confidence – and so reinforces stigma.

We need to educate and inform, so that we can break the vicious cycle of prejudice that runs through public attitudes, media coverage and government priorities. We need to listen and learn from service users and see and involve them as partners and not just as patients. We need to look within ourselves and within our society and acknowledge that we allow an institutionalised stigmatisation to infect our political, social and health systems. Our twin aims must be to convince the public to believe and to convince commission and member states to act. If the public believe, they will put pressure on the European Union (EU) to act. If the EU acts, they will make public belief possible.

We need to look into the eyes of people with mental health problems. When we do, we see reflected back the confusion of emotions and thoughts. We see the fear and worry. We see the tears of frustration and despair. But we also see the hope – the hope that we will listen; that we will understand; that we will care; that we will act; that we can help.

CHAPTER 13

Mental health in Europe: the wider challenge

MICHAEL HOWLETT and CHARLES KAYE

A CASE OF BANANAS

A few items of news about the influence of the European Union (EU) on the domestic affairs of member states, chosen at random on the same day, are instructive in showing us how powerful (or meddling and intrusive, depending on your point of view) Europe has become. Will Hutton, writing in the *The Observer*,[1] claimed that the EU's landmark deal in March 2007 on carbon controls was 'arguably the most important since its foundation 50 years ago'. In the literary section of *The Sunday Telegraph*,[2] Mark Sanderson celebrates the EU's Unfair Commercial Practices Directive, which had to be in force in member states by December 2007, and which will make it illegal for people to write fake reviews of their own books (or of those of their friends). Of course, the fishing industry throughout Europe has felt the effects of the EU's Common Fisheries Policy for many years and recent media stories have described the plight of small fishing boats based in the UK which have already caught their full quota of cod with nine months of the year still to run.[3] Fish caught in excess of any EU-driven quotas have to be thrown back. In the UK, some EU directives have taken on an almost mythical status over time – such as those on the curves of cucumbers and the bends of bananas (bananas must be 'free from malformation or abnormal curvature'[4]) – but in the main, the influence of the EU is real and tangible. As if to celebrate this – and its increasing size – it is reported that the EU plans to open a 'grandiose new "embassy" in London' in 2008, 'just a stone's throw from parliament'.[5]

The EU now has 27 member states, ranging from the UK and the Netherlands in the west to Lithuania, Slovenia, Estonia, Romania and Bulgaria to the east. The size of the Union is expected to increase after 2010, with the accession of Croatia and Turkey. Thereafter, the remaining Balkan states (Macedonia, Albania, Bosnia and Herzegovina, Montenegro, Serbia and Kosovo) are expected to join. By 2020, the EU could have 35 member states with a population in excess of 500 million people.

EUROVISION: MENTAL HEALTH

As Member of the European Parliament (MEP) John Bowis points out in the previous chapter, there are a number of key flaws in mental health services throughout Europe. These include the inadequacy of community provision, the failure to listen to service users and carers, and chronic underfunding. To address these and other pressing concerns, the European region of the World Health Organization (52 member states) endorsed the Mental Health Declaration for Europe, and the Mental Health Action Plan for Europe, in Helsinki in January 2005. The Helsinki Declaration emphasises in broad terms the need for all countries to move away from institutional care to community-based provision, while the Action Plan is more detailed in setting out the need to tackle stigma, to provide a properly trained professional workforce and to listen to the views of patients and carers.

The Helsinki Declaration and Action Plan led to the EU Commission's publishing a Green Paper on mental health in 2005,[6] followed by a period of consultation which ended in May 2006. A number of key findings inform the Green Paper's strategy, which is to concentrate on mental health promotion, social inclusion and civil liberties:

➤ one in four people experience at least one significant episode of mental illness during their lives; in the course of any one year, 18.4 million people in the EU are estimated to suffer from major depression

➤ nearly 60 000 EU citizens commit suicide each year – more than the annual deaths from road traffic accidents or HIV/AIDS – and nearly ten times this number attempt suicide

➤ the economic costs of mental illness to society are substantial, with some estimates putting them at between 3% and 4% of GDP in EU member states

➤ in some member states, up to 85% of funding on mental health is spent on maintaining institutional care

➤ throughout the EU, there is little specific focus on services for children and older people.

The European Parliament's Report in 2006 on the Green Paper (Rapporteur: John Bowis) proposed a motion for a resolution on improving the mental health of the EU population. It is a lengthy and worthy report which, among other things, calls for:

➤ greater commitment to mental health promotion in all member states
➤ recognition of the sizeable differences in mental health expenditure in individual member states
➤ the need to use terminology carefully, such as 'mental ill health', 'mental disorders', 'severe mental illness' and 'personality disorder'
➤ inclusion of people with learning disabilities into any future strategy, based on their experience of stigma, social exclusion, institutionalisation and abuse
➤ a multi-disciplinary, multi-agency response to tackling 'complex mental ill-health situations'
➤ recognition that socially defined images of how girls' and women's bodies should look have an impact on their mental health and well-being, resulting in, among other things, an increase in eating disorders
➤ greater recognition of the connection between discrimination, violence and poor mental health, which 'underlines the importance of combating all forms of violence and discrimination as part of the strategy for the promotion of mental health through prevention'
➤ recognition that any restriction of personal freedoms should be avoided, with particular reference to physical containment, which requires monitoring, verification and vigilance by democratic institutions responsible for upholding individual rights, in order to guard against abuses
➤ calls for the defeat of stigma to be at the heart of any future strategy, for example by establishing annual campaigns on mental health issues in order to combat ignorance and injustice.

And so on. Adoption of the strategy was expected during the spring of 2007. What strikes us about these strategies and proposals is their generalisability, at face value. On the one hand, this is necessarily the case because of the demographics of the EU already described: a vast landmass, with a population approaching 500 million people and widespread differences in terms of political history, culture and economic stability. On the other, however, generalisability should not be taken as an invitation to complacency by those (predominantly western European) nations which boast better standards of care and a more sophisticated and advanced approach. Clearly, these are standards which offer possibilities for all EU countries, west and east, according to the levels at which they are interpreted and addressed. That there is considerable unmet need in Europe is evidenced by a recent study of the epidemiology of mental disorders in Belgium, France, Germany, Italy, the Netherlands and Spain (i.e. western European member states), which found that 31% of the adult population had an unmet need for mental healthcare.[7]

The question is how effective can a pan-European mental health strategy be when it is directed at countries as far apart as Sweden, the UK, the Netherlands, France and Italy on the one hand, and Greece, Turkey, Croatia, Slovakia, Bulgaria and Romania on the other? Can the EU do anything more than make the right noises and gestures concerning mental health provision throughout Europe? Will it, for example, issue directives and establish an inspectorate (or, indeed, a European Observatory on Mental Health, creating, for example, a proactive partnership between member states and the World Health Organization?[8]), so that general ideals and principles can be turned into specific policies? The problem is that there is currently a split between community-focused provision and the institution-based management of mentally ill people, which is fundamentally a split between west and east. The problem is made considerably more complex by recent trends in many western European countries revealing an increase in the use of insitutional care in the west (particularly the use of forensic beds), as well as rising prison populations.[9] And a brief overview of some of the more scandalous practices in institutional care which have recently emerged from new member, accession or candidate states suggests that, in terms of mental health provision, and while clearly it can sponsor reform, the EU faces significant challenges if it is to effect real change in the clinical practice, social care and experiences of highly vulnerable people now coming to its attention.

CAGE BEDS

The difficulties we allude to which face the European Commission as it celebrates its 50th year are illustrated by evidence which has emerged in recent years of the abuse of patients in psychiatric institutions in member states which have accession status, or which have become new members. In 2003 the Mental Disability Advocacy Center (MDAC), based in Budapest, published its research into the use of cage beds in what were then four accession countries: the Czech Republic, Hungary, Slovakia and Slovenia. These countries now enjoy full membership the EU. The report[10] revealed the routine use of cage beds to restrain patients – people with severe intellectual disabilities, the elderly with dementia and mentally disordered people – as a substitute for adequate staffing, or as a punishment. The European Committee for the

Prevention of Torture describes one kind of cage bed as measuring 2.08 m by 0.93 m and being covered 'with a strong net, fixed on a tubular metal structure 1.26 m in height [and] an articulated opening with a padlock'. The MDAC found several types of cage bed in use in its study. The use of cage beds, in some individual cases for years, is a far cry from the more enlightened and ideal standards which have been set elsewhere in the EU, that patients should be treated in the least restrictive setting and in accordance with their human rights; their use is also in stark contrast to the principles which inform the EU's approach, and which are listed above.

Under pressure from the European Commission, some of it led by John Bowis MEP, ministers of health in the Czech Republic and Hungary announced bans on the use of cage beds in 2004. In Slovakia, however, the ban only extends to their use in social care homes, but not in psychiatric hospitals.

TURKEY

Turkey is an accession country and is likely to join the EU in 2010. Judging by recent reports into its treatment of psychiatric patients, there are substantial and significant reforms required before it can be said to meet even basic human requirements. Mental Disability Rights International (MDRI), based in Washington, DC, published a report in 2005[11] which described excessive use of electro-convulsive therapy in Turkish psychiatric institutions, including its use on children as young as nine, unmodified by muscle relaxants or anaesthesia, and the improper use of restraints and seclusion. It also found children 'emaciated from starvation'. The report drew attention to 'inhuman and degrading conditions of confinement [which] are widespread throughout the Turkish mental health system'. People 'are subjected to treatment practices that are tantamount to torture'. A *Sunday Times* report[12] quotes one of the investigators as finding, 'A little girl, who looked to be about two years old, [who] was crying and squirming in her crib. A full bottle of formula was lying in the corner of her crib, just out of reach. I watched for over an hour and no one came to feed her. She would have had nothing if I hadn't helped her.' The absence of community-based provision in Turkey has increased pressure on institutions such as the one described and this imbalance appears to have the status of government policy. The Commission on the Enlargement of the EU has stated that it is monitoring the position of vulnerable groups in candidate countries. A subsequent MDRI report was published in 2006 which graphically illustrates the appalling conditions in which infants and children with disabilities are kept in psychiatric institutions in Romania.[13]

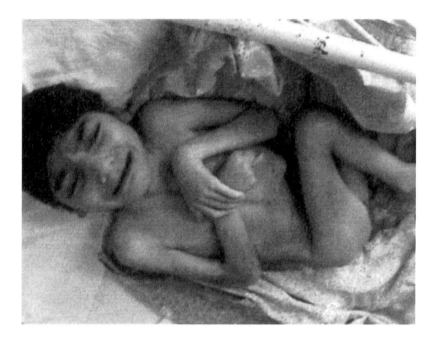

FIGURE 13.1 Hidden suffering: a child in the psychiatric facility in Braila, Romania. *Source:* Mental Disability Rights International, www.mdri.org. Reproduced with permission.

GREEK LESSONS

Greece joined the EU in 1981 and the development of its mental health services since then should inspire cautious optimism, given the challenges faced and those that lie ahead with more recent accessions. Until 1980, mental health services in Greece were totally inadequate to meet the health needs of the population. Shamed into action by scandals such as that discovered on the island of Leros, where 'patients' who weren't even mentally ill were discovered chained and naked in the local psychiatric hospital, and aided by a special EEC regulation which provided the necessary financial support, the Greek Government implemented a wide-ranging programme of reforms. In 1981 there was only one psychiatric unit in a general hospital and six mental health centres. By 1996 these had increased to 30 units (with 321 beds) and 24 mental health centres. Further hospital-based units now offer outpatient and consultation-liaison services. A 10-year plan was agreed in 1997 and continued the programme of deinstitutionalisation in the context of developing primary care and rehabilitation services. Additional programmes focused on developing services for children and older people.

The experience of Greece shows what can done over time, with the support of the EU's financial and regulatory strengths, as well as its oversight. We can go so far as to consider Greece as an exemplar in terms of reforms which are tangible in the wake of a less than satisfactory history. The lesson of Greece is that joining the EU brings with it real responsibilities and commitments, some of which may be culturally and politically counter-intuitive. Given the EU's vision for the future of 'our' mental health services, there is every reason to believe that (from this perspective, at least) membership of this group and this union is preferable to isolation.

THE CHALLENGE AHEAD

'The EU has more platforms than the central station in Brussels.'[14]

The Green Paper proposes a European Platform on Mental Health which will bring together key stakeholders in mental health and public policy to drive the strategy forwards. In spite of a generally agreed consensus about objectives, however, evidence suggests that reform in this critical area of social policy is slow, and real change is hampered by a range of factors that are clearly not the sole responsibility of individual Health ministries: tackling poverty and reducing deprivation is paramount, as the links between economic growth and the economic impact of mental illness are well established (*see* David McDaid's chapter in this book). There is also the political and moral responsibility incumbent upon all member states to provide services in accordance with human rights legislation, to which each member state subscribes on joining the EU. This is not simply a case of the more advanced western democracies waiting for others to 'catch up'. For example, some of the criticisms levelled at the UK's recent proposals to reform mental health law focus on their compatibility with the Human Rights Act. Proponents of reform also point to the need for more individual freedom in service provision and access to care, and greater choice for patients within this context. We need to recognise that there are many objectives still to be realised, and deficiencies which need to be addressed. So, while the rhetoric in the UK may have graduated to levels of sophistication not enjoyed elsewhere in Europe, the principles remain broadly the same and, as we have suggested, there is no room for complacency.

We have seen in our snapshot of Europe how the EU has responded to scandals on a country-by-country basis. That the EU appears to rely upon reports by non-government organisations, the voluntary sector and the media is a concern. Information mapping about the extent of unmet need and what is going on in all member states is one of its greatest challenges. With countries in the east at radically different stages of the 'post-asylum' era in the institutional sense, and struggling in the west to cope with the mental health needs of thousands of refugees seeking asylum in the political sense, the need for some kind of centralised pan-European monitoring system is pressing, yet there is currently no formal infrastructure within Europe with a specific mental health remit. It has taken 50 years to develop a strategy and a platform for mental health. Demographically, politically and culturally, as we have seen, the EU has undergone radical changes in that time and has brought upon itself greater challenges than ever. We can only hope its ambitions for mental health promotion and service provision can be effectively realised within such a diverse, complex and sometimes retrogressive framework. While the pace and rhythm of change remain slow, there is some justification for cautious optimism.

REFERENCES

1 Hutton W. How Europe can save the world. London: *The Observer*; 11 March 2007.
2 Sanderson M. Literary life. London: *The Sunday Telegraph*; 11 March 2007.
3 Booker C. EU quotas sink Britain's small fishing boats. London: *The Sunday Telegraph*; 11 March 2007.
4 Commission Regulation (EC) No. 2257/94.
5 Smith N. EU 'to waste' £1 m a year on stately London embassy. London: *The Sunday Telegraph*; 11 March 2007.
6 European Commission. *Improving the mental health of the population. Towards a strategy on mental health for the European Union.* Strasbourg: Com (2005) 484.
7 Alonso J, Codony M, Kovess V, *et al.* Population level of unmet need for mental healthcare in Europe. *Br J Psychiatry.* 2007; **190**: 299–306.
8 Wahlbeck K, McDaid D. Enhancing the policy relevance of mental health related research in Europe. *Eurohealth.* 2005; **11**(4): 13.
9 Priebe S, Badesconyi A, Fioritti A, *et al.* Reinstitutionalisation in mental health care: comparison of data on service provision from six European coutries. *BMJ.* 2006; **330**: 123–6.
10 Mental Disability Advocacy Center. *Cage Beds: inhuman and degrading treatment in four EU accession countries.* Budapest: Mental Disability Advocacy Center; 2003.
11 Mental Disability Rights International. *Behind Closed Doors: human rights abuses in the psychiatric facilities, orphanages and rehabilitation centers of Turkey.* Washington, DC: Mental Disability Rights International; 2005.
12 Smith N. Child patients starve in Turkey's mental hospitals. London: *The Sunday Times*; 9 October 2005.
13 Mental Disability Rights International. *Hidden and Suffering: Romania's segregation and abuse of infants and children with disabilities.* Washington, DC: Mental Disability Rights International; 2006.
14 Needle C. The EU mental health platform. *Eurohealth.* 2005; **11**(4): 11.

Index